THE
BITTERSWEETNESS
OF DIABETES

Also written by Cheryl Lynn Kantzer Crane:

Alaska Bound On The Cheryl Lynn: A Mariner's Rhyming Log

My personal journey through
discovery, recovery, and overcoming

THE
BITTERSWEETNESS
OF DIABETES

Cheryl Lynn Kantzer Crane

Illustrated by Jim Greenwald

Foreword by Scot Brower, MD

The author may be contacted by email:
larrydcrane@aol.com

ISBN 978-1-935089-17-9

Acacia Publishing, Inc.
Phoenix, Arizona

www.acaciapublishing.com

Printed and bound in the United States of America

Disclaimer

The author of this book does not dispense medical advice or prescribe the use of any techniques as a form of treatment for any physical or medical problems without the advice of a physician, either directly or indirectly. The intent of the author is only to offer information about how it is to personally experience living with brittle diabetes, and to help you in your quest for emotional well-being, good health, and not allow diabetes to steal your dreams or life. In the event you use any of the information in this book for yourself, which is your constitutional right, the author and the publisher assume no responsibility for your actions. The mention of companies, organizations, or authorities in this publication does not imply endorsement by the publisher, nor does mention of specific companies, organizations, or authorities in the publication imply that they endorse the publication.

Acknowledgements

There are many people including family, friends, medical practitioners, and complete strangers I wish to thank for helping me in the writing of this book. Their patience, added support, and suggestions made a valuable impact in all aspects up to getting it published.

I would especially like to thank my California cousin, Tom Helman, who was an insightful book doctor, spending many hours with me over the phone and emailing. He was instrumental in fine-tuning, probing, and dissecting my book, shedding new light and stretching my mind to see other ways to approach.

I would like to give further special thanks to Dr. Allen Sussman, M.D. for taking time out from his busy schedule to give me his keen insight, thoughts, and attitudes.

I would also sincerely like to thank Dr. Scot Brower, M.D., for his input, besides his skillful, steady, laser-gun hands during my eye surgeries.

I am further indebted to nurse Denise Bakke, for her willingness to take the time to give me her comments and viewpoints. My neighbor and friend, Aleni Mang, was most helpful in her detailed critique, adding to the flow of my book. Many additional thanks to my friend, Cindy Louie, for her scrutinizing my work, focusing more on some of the smaller details and her constant moral support at all stages of my book. I appreciated finding Leslie Hoffman, who was willing to edit my rhyming book, and I am very grateful for the illustrating talents of Jim Greenwald.

I owe many heartfelt thanks to my computer gurus, Dayna Evensen and Janet West, for sharing their computer wisdom in lessening my anxiety in our computerized world. I enjoyed thoroughly and wish to thank the Sun City West Writer's Group and their leader, Ethel Neidoff, who is a fellow rhymer. I looked forward to all of the advice and critiques that were generously given each month.

Additional thanks to my 'Heart' Mother, Isabel Mays VanValey, for her honest critique and a mother's encouragement. Last, but not least, I would like to express my gratitude to my husband, Larry D. Crane, for his steady, loving support, chauffeuring, using more than his share of culinary and domestic talents, and listening with at least one ear. Living with a writer with diabetes isn't always easy, especially during the stillness of the night, when the lights flash on, not due to low sugars, but to jot down my fleeting thoughts before I lose them.

I dedicate this book to:

All of you who have kept me on the road
to wellness, to living,
Thank you for all of your support and thoughtfulness,
and for all of your giving.

My husband, Larry Dean Crane:

Occasionally, I do need to touch him
to see if my husband is for real.
He is one of the best things that has happened
in my life – to me he's ideal.

To my dad in his memory, C. Jack Kantzer:

He's guiding, watching, and protecting
me from far above.
He was my best friend; I cherish our times together
and the sharing of his love.

My 'Heart' parents—
The late James Nugent Mays
and Isabel Lorene Mays VanValey:

Who welcomed me into their home
to help my dad raise me when I was three,
with their continual support, love, and caring ways,
I do feel lucky.

Table of Contents

Foreword

Many years ago a young woman walked into my office. She was a juvenile diabetic and she was experiencing decreased vision. This young woman was Cheryl Crane. A careful eye examination revealed that she was suffering from diabetic retinopathy. Specifically, she had a type of retinopathy called Macular Edema. In this condition the diabetes damages the small blood vessels of the retina and causes them to become leaky. As a result, serum leaks out of the blood vessels and into the retina causing it to be wet and thickened from swelling. Unfortunately, a wet retina does not see well. Cheryl was referred to San Francisco to consult with a world authority on the subject, who was using some new laser techniques to treat patients with her problem. Cheryl underwent several laser treatments on both eyes to halt the deterioration of her vision. Ultimately these treatments were successful in drying up her wet retinas and curing her macular edema, but, unfortunately, she was left with decreased and impaired vision.

The real story here, however, is not Cheryl's eye problem or its treatment. The real story is about how Cheryl coped with her loss of vision. In my entire career, I have never had anyone handle such a devastating loss of vision in such a brave and bold fashion. Cheryl refused to accept the fact that she was impaired or disabled. As a result of her attitude she trained and retrained herself to live with her impaired vision. Cheryl developed new skills and new ways of working and playing.

Cheryl continued to teach and work full time. She was an inspiration to her students and fellow teachers. She was well liked by her students, who sensed her strength and accomplishments. At one point when the school district became concerned about safety issues, Cheryl took them on in her typical confrontational style. As a result she was given certain low vision aides and allowed to continue to teach, and did a fine job at it.

Cheryl refused to allow her decreased and impaired vision to limit her life. She was used to having a very active and busy life. She was very athletic and outdoor oriented and was not about to give this all up because of her vision loss. Despite being legally blind with 20/200 visual acuity, Cheryl carried on, continuing all the sports she loved. She water skied in the summer and snow skied in the winter. She hiked, biked and climbed in the mountains. Cheryl and her husband took their boat north to Alaska, fishing and crabbing as they went. I am still not certain how Cheryl has continued to be so active in these demanding sports, but a lot of it is by sheer willpower and her unwillingness to give up.

Cheryl has been an inspiration to me as an ophthalmologist. I cannot remember any patients who have worked harder to carry on a normal life than Cheryl. Despite a significant loss of vision, she has carried on a full and normal life injected with adventure and hard work. She has truly lived her life to the fullest extent. This has not only brought happiness to her and her husband, Larry, but also to her friends, students and fellow teachers. Many have been inspired by her attitude and hard work and as a result they have bettered themselves.

It has been an honor and a privilege to have been allowed to share in Cheryl's medical care. I have enjoyed all of our office visits and have always come away from them with a positive feeling in my heart. I have been awed by Cheryl's ability to make the most of life without ever complaining. She accepted her fate and moved on, accomplishing much and living a very productive and fulfilling life.

Scot Brower, MD
Ophthalmologist

Author's Preface

My symptoms were prevalent, but the disease was undiagnosed for nearly two years. After several months of unquenchable thirst, yeast infections, fatigue, and other symptoms, I turned twenty in 1971. That was the year I discovered that the rest of my life would be framed within the blood sugar range of 80-120. That was the year I began to become a lay-expert on controlling and manipulating my blood sugar level. That was the year I realized all the challenges I would be facing as I left college to make my way in the world were subject to my ability to triumph over this slippery disease: diabetes.

My intent is to offer information regarding how it is to experience living with brittle diabetes and being vision-impaired. I hope to help other diabetics in their quest for emotional well-being and good health, while avoiding the temptation to allow diabetes, its complications, or any other disease to steal one's dreams or life.

When the doctors were diagnosing my mysterious illness, diabetes did not occur to them. I didn't have the usual characteristics such as being genetically prone, young, or past the age of forty.

In addition, I was neither pregnant nor obese, and did not fall in any of the target ethnic groups.

I have experienced the range of emotions that you might suspect as my life has unfolded. But perhaps the most difficult has been reconciling my uncompromising desire to win with the few half victories that I have achieved in trying to conquer diabetes. In the beginning, diabetes was a battle I was not winning. Even with my competitive, fighting spirit, it seemed like I was losing the battle. I was furious that I was the exception to the so-called diabetic rules; I was not the stereotypical diabetic that the medical professionals would read about in a book. I am a brittle diabetic, having fluctuating blood sugars from very low, below 50, to above 300, unrelated to lifestyle inconsistencies and indiscretions.

It took a long time for me to find my smile, think more positively, and be more accepting of my irregularities in trying to manage this disease. I was an active, athletic, young college student, entering the adult world, intending to continue accomplishing a long list of goals. I enjoyed snow skiing, water skiing, running, basketball, volleyball, racquetball, and many other sports. I wanted to keep traveling and further my college education. I liked keeping busy and was reluctant to sit still. The whole world was laid out before me to explore, achieve, and accomplish.

Since a very young age, I was very competitive, focused, and determined to be successful in whatever I set my mind to do. I had this strong need to win and be number one. I strived for perfection and took great pleasure in marking off my accomplished goals. I always fought hard and did my best, whether I won or not. Yet, with diabetes, it was a battle that was getting the best of me. My family knew I was stubborn, determined, bullheaded, and not a quitter; however, diabetes brought these traits out stronger. They did not realize it was the illness and thought it was part of my basic personality. I was following the advice of my doctors, but often, I was an exception to the rules. It did not seem to matter what I did, my diabetes was uncooperative, and it was winning. To my family, it was unclear how hard I was fighting to keep my diabetes under control. I was misread as being belligerent, ornery, and not taking good care of myself. It was a struggle to adapt to this new lifestyle change, my lifelong battle.

After my diagnosis, I tried to win by following the same strategy that had served me so well in the past. I refused to give in to fatigue and physically worked out, at times to my detriment. I attended diabetic school, followed the rules and all of the advice that medical science had given me, but soon realized that this strategy was not working. Unfortunately, being a brittle diabetic, I can have a low blood sugar count, eating the right foods and doing the same activity one day to find those same foods can have a different effect the next day. I can follow all the rules and find myself in a coma being rushed to the hospital by family and friends. Upon recovering, I am once again subjected to the same lecture of the need to follow a proper diet, control my blood sugar levels, and take better care of myself. Frustratingly, I try to convince the medical staff that, no, I haven't been forgetting to self-monitor my blood sugars, abusing my body with improper food, or just not eating at all. I have been a good student, I have been a good strategist, I am just temporarily on a losing team.

I have not given in to the temptation to give up, to sleep away my life within the limitations of fatigue. As you read my book, you will follow me as I have a career as a teacher, travel through Europe, enjoy and sail my R20 sailboat, travel to Alaska in our 41 ft. PT trawler, join the ski patrol, and perform feats of physical challenge to prove to myself that I can lead a normal life. You will also join me in the trips to the hospital, the seven laser surgeries, and experiencing legal blindness. In addition, collapsing across the threshold of my own home so that someone would notice and get me some help.

This book shares with you the many personal challenges and struggles of dealing with the unknown symptoms, managing and controlling a disease that for me was and still is unpredictable, and most importantly, changing my mindset to a more positive outlook. Facing the demands of my health challenges made it more difficult to stay motivated in dealing with so many uncertainties, fearing the unknown and its threatening complications. For me to stay healthy this disease requires firm discipline, effort, energy, and commitment. By putting myself through many physical and mental tests, I found that diabetes and being legally blind was not going to stop me in fulfilling my dreams. Earlier, I was too often misusing my energy by being angry, hateful, and worried about the difficulty in accomplishing my many goals.

Yes, I have adapted with the times and have the latest and the best diabetic treatment equipment that is available to me. I appreciatively wear my insulin pump and eagerly await any new scientific research or opinion I can find, whether it's western medicine or alternative, untraditional medicine. But what has sustained my hope and gotten me through so much has been my family and friends. In 1991, I married my very own EMT (Emergency Medical Technician), a firefighter, whose kindness and understanding are overwhelming. When I have to wake myself up at 2:00 a.m. to check my blood sugar level, there he is, my wonderful soulmate, watching me with concern for my well-being.

I have written this book in rhyme, using couplets, creating my own rhythmic pattern. I find this form allows me to best express myself. Listen for the anger, bitterness, hope, and love that can be expressed in the free-falling process of poetry. Diabetes for me has been unpredictable, not always following the norm, so I have chosen this unique verse to describe it.

Studying metaphysical disciplines and learning to use my latent senses, including my sixth sense, has awakened my intuitive faculties, put me in touch with my inner world, and allowed me to gain more self-understanding. It has offered an alternative view, shedding new light on the health issues and problems in my life. Adversity has not made me stronger; the will to lead my life and achieve my goals has done that. Finding out I could still pursue my interests and challenge myself to learn new ones has given me a more positive attitude. Now, I can find humor in most of my diabetic and low vision episodes. My life has taken a turn and I am still fighting battles, but with less anger and hatred, and with more understanding. I am in control; the diabetes is not in control of me. It was not easy getting to this point.

Cheryl Lynn Kantzer Crane

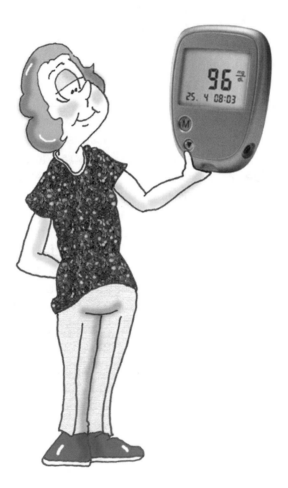

Chapter 1

Some, like me, are sensitive to insulin
  and are categorized as being brittle.
We have our fair share of difficulties
  in keeping our unstable sugars in the middle.

In the beginning, most health practitioners
  thought all diabetics were the textbook kind.
This includes today's medical insurances,
  who I want to give a piece of my mind!

Some, like me, are sensitive to insulin
  and are categorized as being brittle.
We have our fair share of difficulties
  in keeping our unstable sugars in the middle.

With irregular blood sugars, I'm constantly worrying,
  is it going up or down?
Silently wondering, if I am in need of a sugar boost,
  will there be someone around?

My blood sugars are unrelated
  to lifestyle inconsistencies and indiscretions.
They'll fluctuate from below fifty to above three hundred,
  not following my directions.

Why must I deal with having erratic glucose levels?
    It seems to be the norm for me.
There must be a Higher reason.
    It's out of my hands or control; I truthfully do believe.

My dear doctor, my endocrinologist comments,
    "Why do you think it is going down?
It could be on its way up," as I listen attentively,
    eyeing him with a doubtful frown.

Juggling this sugary balancing act is testing me,
    but I won't lose; I will win!
The universe knows I am strong, persistent,
    and bullheaded: it is dealing with Cheryl Lynn.

On one occasion before bed, I checked
    my blood sugar level at 9:30 that night.
I said with some fear, "Hey, I'm a 98.
    Do you think I'm safe?" I love having it just right.

My husband replies suspiciously, faltering in doubt,
    "We just never really know with you."
This is an ongoing struggle, which much to my disappointment,
    I am finding so true.

Whether my blood sugars are soaring or too low,
    I seldom receive an obvious clue.
These subtle warnings are baffling, since I'm unable
    to prepare myself in what to do.

My incredulous sugars do make it trying
    in noting a suggestive guiding cue.
I wish I would get more recognizable signs,
    Instead, at times, of only getting a few.

Thus, after all these years in having to manage
    and live with diabetes for so long,
It's become increasingly harder to notice both low
    or high symptoms. They've left me; they're gone.

It's a nauseous, sickening feeling
    when my sugars reach a hyperglycemic state.
When they are climbing and rising too high
    and they are not noticed until it is much too late.

Plus, it's frustrating dipping into hypoglycemia,
    being low isn't my goal.
Not even the slightest hint, that my body needs
    orange juice, Starburst, or to grab the sugar bowl.

Rarely am I warned by symptoms to insulin reactions:
    sweat, shakes, or slurring my speech.
Deep within my consciousness, I must hope
    someone's alert, able, or sugar is in arm's reach.

It's very confusing after I've just checked
    my sugar level or have eaten a meal.
It is teaching me to think beyond logic,
    to learn to be intuitive in how I feel.

Every illness, medical problem, or disease
    has a lesson for us all to learn.
Most likely, this is one of the many I've chosen
    as I am passing through this life's sojourn.

There are times I have blood sugars as low as the thirties;
    I am in a stuporous state.
Then other times for some reason,
    I'm able to do my activities and communicate.

Even though there's some confusion and unclear thinking,
    I'm not a hundred percent fully there.
My unfocused mind will wander off
    as I will begin to get the diabetic blank stare.

With great indomitable effort,
    I will keep driving myself harder and persevere.
Despite the fact my energy level has dropped,
    descending down to its sluggish lowest gear.

Sheer determination, stubbornness, and perhaps,
    orneriness keep me pushing myself
To finish whatever task I am presently doing
    before seeking any sugar help.

It's not only just with blood sugars, whether they are
    too low to function, normal, or high.
I was born with this relentless inner drive
    not to give up, but to make sure I try, try, try.

Thank goodness for my intuitive husband, Larry,
    who is very alert in catching many.
He'd be rich, living a dreamy, luxurious life,
    if for each one he received a penny.

My thought processes slow down becoming confused.
    My physical body is hard to move.
My husband takes close note of my abnormal behavior
    as I am not in the Cheryl Lynn groove.

I'm aware my guardian angel is not perfect.
    He cannot catch all the warnings.
I do appreciate the ones he does catch,
    especially the ones in the early mornings.

I admit, it's not all easy living with me
    when he suggests my blood sugar is low.
Instead of testing, I'll argue, get irritable,
    and be rude; I bluntly refuse to show.

He is in tune with my body rhythms
    and understands I'm not my speedy self, but slow.
I'll defy and resist, while trying to drive
    my bullheaded self forward, staying on the go.

It's difficult for me to think clearly through,
    or to act, or speak, like I normally do.
Thus, this helps my husband to clue in that
    my blood sugars might possibly be slightly askew.

In addition, there are times when I believe
    he's being insensitive and being mean.
With such furious intensity, I try, but am unable
    to push forward with full steam.

This causes us more cantankerous quarreling
    until my blood sugar level is checked.
Then, as much as I hate to admit in being wrong,
    most of the time, my husband is correct.

Since a child, I have hated to lose, always needing
    to be triumphant, win, and be right.
Whether it's a heated argument, a cause,
    or playing a simple game of cards, I will fight.

My husband voices his opinion,
    "She often can make it difficult for me, she's tough.
It seems like in everything she does, my wife will not give up.
    Even if she breaks, she won't slough!"

5

Such personality traits have helped me
in dealing with my diabetic brittleness.
I am grateful it's in my genes for my diabetic life
has been filled with bittersweetness.

I'd be dishonest if I said
being a diabetic is easy and relaxing.
It can be most exasperating, tiring,
and on my mind and body, very taxing.

This sugary balancing act is a constant worry
and does weigh heavily on my mind.
Do I have enough juice, Starburst, or the right snacks,
and are they in easy reach for the right time?

Or when I'm sleepy and I want to fall fast asleep,
will I without an assist wake up?
Or will my worrisome husband find me
in a diabetic coma with my mouth seized shut?

How's my blood sugar level? Is it rebounding,
bouncing around from too high to too low?
I can't stand not knowing these unpredictable,
indistinct symptoms – I have this need to know.

Can I safely do this activity or this exercise?
Do I need to check again?
My pierced fingers are sore and are aching.
I must avoid infection. They need some time to mend.

I fear running out of strips. My insurance won't budge.
Have I been using too many?
I check my blood sugar at least six times a day.
Will my allotted monthly supply be plenty?

Do I have enough of my supplies for traveling
    or for even a short daily trip?
There are fleeting moments when I'm utterly
    exhausted, and I honestly don't give a rip.

Once in awhile, I want to be free
    in not taking all of my extra supplies with me.
How relieved to eliminate one less bag, thinking
    this is only a short, quick shopping spree.

Will my overprotective hubby ever join me
    in slacking off, in letting me be?
I do try to see it from his point of view, and keep hoping
    there's a chance for both of us to agree.

Naturally, it never fails. I do need something
    when I do not have a single thing.
I then must brace against his explosive emotions erupting
    as my ears begin to ring!

Each morning after waking up, I faithfully
    first check my blood sugar, which sets the tone.
It makes it at times rather difficult to plan for the day
    because it is always unknown.

When, what, and how much am I allowed to eat,
    checking before or after I've exercised.
I don't want to feel at all weak. I want
    my mind, body, and spirit to feel reenergized.

Whether it is to my liking or not,
    my blood sugar results rule the rest of my day.
I need to keep a watchful eye and stay on top of things,
    whether I am at rest or at play.

I struggle not to look at the negative side of things,
    or allow it to get me down.
I try to focus more on the positive,
    as every negative can be turned around.

As we need to believe, every negative
    has a positive, a much nicer sound.
We might have to open our eyes somewhat further,
    but eventually the good can be found.

Here is a small example of what I did once
    when I had a tough year teaching junior high.
I would force myself to zero in on more positive thoughts,
    not allowing myself to cry.

I would take caution in guarding against
    my energy from being totally consumed,
As a disruptive troublemaker made his grand entrance,
    waltzing lively into my classroom.

It is stretching, however, I would say wordlessly,
    he sure tied his shoes nicely today.
It is a brand new day, hoping he will not give me
    any more flak. He will choose to obey.

Once I became fully conscious of my situation,
    accepting my limitations,
I was freer to maximize my full potential
    with more reasonable expectations.

As I've been learning to accept my limitations
    in my own personal universe,
I'm finally realizing the deeper meaning,
    and then, diabetes is not such a curse.

It's my spiritual life path, my fated journey,
    which I have previously chosen.
I do wonder why at times, this karmic destiny
    I am in the midst of and have woven.

What are my hidden lessons, I can't imagine.
    I have chosen to be legally blind.
Yet, it is my fate, therefore, out of my control,
    so now, I must accept and treat myself kind.

Here's what was written in a Chinese fortune cookie
    which fascinated me.
"The beginning of wisdom is to desire it,"
    which I find true and strongly do agree.

Fear causes limitations, blocking me,
    so it is important to learn to love myself.
Love enhances and aids my healing, bringing me
    deserving happiness with much better health.

Life has been tough in discovering my true self.
    We all must accept who we truly are.
Not allowing anyone or anything to trap us
    or browbeat us with an iron bar.

Others always seem to tell their diabetic horror stories,
    which I don't wish to hear.
We, diabetics, are already quite aware,
    and that is what I deep down secretly fear.

Yes, it is true; my once 20/20 vision
    is impaired due to my diabetes.
More reason to keep a sound body and mind
    and not just by relying on eating Wheaties.

Toxic thoughts can dim my inner and outer light,
    not allowing myself to shine as bright.
I must keep surrounding myself with those who'll
    support and heal me with their positive white light.

Treatments of some diseases are grim
    and as trying as the actual diagnosis.
Thus, I'm blessed, since after treatment
    one feels better following a diabetes prognosis.

The bottom line is, I am just a normal person
    in dealing with a chronic disease.
Perhaps, not according to how society views it,
    but this is what I, Cheryl Lynn, see.

Chapter II

*I was driven to fight more as the diabetic symptoms
    progressively became worse.
My thick skull could not recognize the
    physical messages or the ones from the universe.*

When I was a college sophomore, I was
    unsuspectingly relieved, but was deeply stunned.
The medical field discovered I had diabetes.
    I thought my life was over and done.

This particular stressful day was marked
    as a crisis, one that is unforgettable.
Wondering what lies ahead for me and
    inspiring much fear, hoping I'll be capable.

Actually, I didn't have much of a clue
    about this chronic disease, diabetes.
I had heard one must eliminate sugar
    from one's diet, especially all sweet goodies.

Thinking back, I realized, that I had endured
    the aggravating symptoms for quite awhile.
It took a couple of years for the correct diagnosis,
    which certainly has changed my lifestyle.

I believed I suffered from all listed symptoms
    that are found in a diabetic book;
Visited doctors, not only at home, but while
    studying in Germany to take a look.

My first year as an aspiring college freshman
    could have been more pleasurable.
I even had experienced a few symptoms
    while in high school that were immeasurable.

I thought settling in had physically drained me
    as I missed my language placement test.
Sleeping soundly through my alarm, I wasn't aware
    my tired body needed more than rest.

Despite the many symptoms, I still made
    the Varsity volleyball team my freshman year.
Not realizing how much easier it could have been,
    as I was always in a sluggish gear.

Dealing with severe leg cramps and having
    great difficulty keeping wide-wake in class,
It didn't ever seem to matter how early I went to bed,
    my sleepy eyes would not last.

My unquenchable, fierce thirst was so irritating,
    putting me on the edge of despair.
There didn't seem to be a satisfying liquid to help,
    at least one that I was aware.

I would desperately line up juice, pop,
    all available dorm drinks to experiment.
Taking only a few sips told me I was setting myself up
    for a big disappointment.

No stomach growls as I had no interest
    beyond quenching my thirst, thus, no appetite.
All food, dorm or not, was not appealing.
    I'd pick at it, occasionally, taking a bite.

I was beside myself in the numerous attempts
    for a quick cure, not knowing from what.
If I'd vanished off the earth, would someone
    remember me with the flower, the Forget-Me-Not?

When summer came, I rushed home to partake
    in my sister's wedding, then off on an airplane.
I wasn't home long enough for anyone to notice
    these symptoms or for me to complain.

As I attended summer school in Germany,
    the bothersome symptoms continued on.
Today, it's merely impossible to fathom
    how I suffered unknowingly for so long.

I always focused on keeping myself in top shape,
    feeling strong and confidently sure.
I still dealt with an insatiable thirst, yeast infections,
    tired, and my eyes began to blur.

Having sunshiny weather, I unjustly blamed
    my weakening eyes on seeing heat waves,
Feeling disempowered and so fatigued,
    returning promptly to bed was what my body craved.

My desire to be in peak shape was contrary
    to my body's resistance to run.
To reenergize myself further, I swam pool laps
    and laid in the healing warmth of the sun.

The local kids were a partial distraction
    and amused in helping me with my German.
Despite my ill health, speaking and learning German
    filled me with high spirits, creating some fun.

Further attempts to quench my endless thirst,
    my girlfriend and I would share a liter of pop.
However, once again, it never seemed like enough
    or would do the trick; the thirst did not stop.

My ongoing yeast infections led me
    to another clinic for some medication.
This time to be sure, I asked for some help
    with the medical German to English translation.

Determined to stay in shape, I shared the track
    with the German army as the sun would rise.
No matter what I tried to do, I felt rotten.
    This was unlike me and took me by surprise.

I was driven to fight more as the diabetic symptoms
    progressively became worse.
My thick skull could not recognize the
    physical messages or the ones from the universe.

One night driving by a hospital, I was feeling poorly,
    which still to this day haunts me.
My Higher Self was pleading, Stop! Please take me.
    I couldn't act, despite the urging, silent plea.

Unfortunately, the words were never voiced.
    They kept racing madly through my powerless thoughts.
I just could not get myself to speak aloud.
    It was as if my vocal chords were tied in knots.

As my mom hugged me when I returned,
    she smelled the sweet fragrance like Juicy Fruit gum.
Thinking nothing of it but its nice aroma,
    not knowing it's a high blood sugar symptom.

Eager in returning to school in the fall,
    I decided not to spend much time in Kent.
I first wanted to see a doctor from home
    who was highly recommended, then, off I went.

Having the frame of mind of always keeping myself fit,
    healthy, and my young body sound,
Didn't help very much, or if I had stayed home longer,
    perhaps the symptoms might have been found.

I was haunted by this repeated vision
    of passing out cold on the campus's main square;
Being hauled off by medics as the heavy feelings lifted,
    having no more worries or care.

My obvious, undiagnosed symptoms
    were becoming worse, not fully understanding why.
Nevertheless, I dug my heels in deeper
    to keep fighting to stay unknowingly alive.

As I pushed myself to sprint down the soccer field,
    it felt as if I was in slow motion.
It took too much effort for me. I was imagining
    and dreaming for a secret potion.

Plus, I constantly had the urge to go to the bathroom.
    The frequency was annoying.
This strong need was as often as every couple of minutes.
    This I was not enjoying.

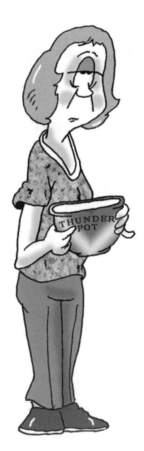

As I'd rise off the toilet seat, the feeling remained.
    My body still signaled me to go.
Even if I sat longer, it didn't help.
    I needed a thunder pot, keeping one in tow.

To gain some extra sleeping time,
    I took a required class at home via our TV.
Hence, my days were still uncommonly tiring,
    so my cleverness didn't seem to help me.

My sights were set to be a ski instructor.
    My ongoing thirst led me to eating snow.
My body was downright miserable on the slopes,
    besides my bladder's frequent urge to flow.

Test results show
    I'm diabetic. Oh, No!

At last, after another doctor visit,
    he had taken a long overdue blood test.
He noticed exceptional high blood sugars,
    presenting a clue why I'm not feeling my best.

He said I needed to see a surgeon right away,
    not comprehending exactly why.
This upsetting phone call didn't make any sense to me,
    or to my dad, "Oh, dear me, oh my!"

Researching with the assistance of my dad's friends,
    Dad found at that time the best place to be.
My entire life was taking a gigantic, whirlwind turn
    and was now moving rapidly.

My stress was soaring high, as my life wasn't running smoothly,
   difficult to find some peace.
I wasn't aware yet how stress significantly affects sugars,
   to increase or decrease.

It wasn't helping when I was trying to get permission
   to take my finals early.
One professor would not allow and added to my stress.
   He was being a little surly.

Until the Dean of Students, my savior, came to my assistance,
   politely stepping in,
The narrow-minded professor did lose this one battle,
   for I, Cheryl Lynn, did tiredly win.

Too many battles, strain, and tension
   added to my already stressed out, weakened body.
Now wondering, was it stress or my unstable, brittle sugars,
   making me feel so shoddy?

It wasn't too smart in regulating
   when I'd eat a whole candy bar when I felt low.
I was stressed not having control and used the excuse
   to eat sugar since it was a no-no.

It angered me more, since I could not truly enjoy it
   while in this low sugary state.
With the upsetting weight gain and bouncing sugars,
   I still did not care at first how much I ate.

I had this strong desire in wanting to run, but which way,
   searching for extra protection.
I had many short and long-range goals I must achieve.
   I did not like my new life's direction.

I was relieved, my medical puzzle was figured out,
    but still not understanding a lot.
Anxious to learn, but still a dispirited soul,
    so many unknowns kept thickening the plot.

There were so many questions with very few answers.
    I needed to find out what I could.
Partially aware and scared of what I can or cannot do,
    attempting to do what I should.

Through experience, I learned to refrain from
    mentioning my unhealthy situation.
I'd hear frightening stories of families
    with kidney failure, blindness, or amputation.

With unsettling emotions, I need to stay realistic
    in dealing with my health troubles.
Whether fears are real or imagined,
    I can't live in fantasy or idealistic bubbles.

I wondered with this major interruption,
    how do I keep grounded? Is it possible?
Managing this unwanted sugar-forbidden disease
    seemed to me to be impossible.

Meanwhile, the doctor suggested getting further help
    from the college's infirmary.
This was all so overwhelming, with finals
    and not feeling well, being physically weary.

In my opinion, they gave me the wrong book to read
    to learn more about diabetes.
It described how eons ago they drank their own urine
    to heal and other tasteless goodies.

Of course, I wasn't the most jovial person,
    even when friends tried to humor or tease.
The book frightened me. Yet, gaining knowledge
    is beneficial for this newly diagnosed disease.

My kind aunt, who was a nurse,
    also had prescribed a magazine on diabetic news.
It was hard for me to read only the neutral parts
    like recipes without feeling the blues.

I know I must learn and keep informed,
    getting educated is a valuable thing.
However, the more I read, the more disturbing stories I'd hear,
    not liking this sound or ring.

My pancreas isn't producing the hormone insulin,
    or obviously enough.
My blood sugars would keep climbing out of control,
    especially from eating any foodstuff.

Therefore, the physician had given me some pills,
    but said they most likely won't do the job.
He figured this would be a gentler approach,
    knowing how I could easily begin to sob.

He said stomach acids would most likely destroy
    the pill before it could do any good.
Could a simple small pill, Ornase, bring me back
    to my ol' healthy me; what is the likelihood?

The dreaded painful insulin shots were inevitable.
    It was time for me to learn.
The school infirmary had me practicing on oranges,
    causing me to squirm with much concern.

Changing my ingrained eating habits
  and finding sugar-free food was not an easy task,
Besides, telling a college student there's no more drinking,
  not even up skiing with my flask.

I was not aware before of how much sugar I ate,
  it was found in most everything.
I couldn't even spread jam on my toast
  or munch on snacks while studying in the evening.

What a distraction from my college studies,
  as my school mind now worries, wanders, and drifts.
I will profit from following my instructions,
  hoping in the near future my spirit lifts.

More do's and don'ts to learn;
  I need answers to my diabetic concerns.

Attending school to help conquer and learn
  about diabetes has finally arrived.
It'll be a mighty long week. My parents and I
  want to be able to say, I have survived.

I was still feeling shattered and devastated
  with the shocking news of this diagnosis.
My brain is on overload. I am feeling depleted.
  Will I be learning through osmosis?

My emotions are unstable. They're being blocked.
  How much will I be able to take in?
How crystal clear will my thoughts be, as I am holding
  too many of my fears tightly within?

Will I be able to concentrate, keeping my ears open
    about my new health concerns?
This chapter of my life is terrifying,
    making me feel restless as another page turns.

Because I was refusing to stay overnight,
    I was, therefore, transported in each day.
I was being my stubborn, ornery, self.
    Yet, I wanted to feel better, so what can I say.

Most of my notes were written in German.
    I kept alone in my fast changing, angry world.
With such mental and physical exhaustion,
    I dreamed to lie in the fetal position, curled.

The staff was flabbergasted as my thighs and arms
        were looking like a challenging ski slope.
With too many lumps and hollows like bumpy ski moguls,
    It depressed me, causing me to mope.

They were curious where, who and how
    I was instructed in giving my insulin shots.
Not knowing any better, I'll now need new methods
    besides finding other injection spots.

Apprehensive to use my tender stomach,
    I'll need to find my positive attitude.
Realizing there really isn't a choice, I just hope
    I have the inner strength and fortitude.

It was surprising to many in how quickly
    it all happened, all within a month's span.
I'd need to clothe my body, so I was unrecognizable
    as a woman or a man.

In fact, my dad blamed my dented limbs
on my mom, who occasionally gave me my shot.
She was more hurt than angry and said, "Never again!"
The atmosphere was tense and boiling hot.

This led me to volunteer for a research group,
thinking it might have been the insulin.
My lumpy skin vanished after several years,
now gratefully looking like it had once been.

This study made me self-conscious and ill at ease,
when pictures were snapped of my deformities,
Adding more anxiety to shot-giving,
fearful in creating more abnormalities.

The results for this uncommon problem were unclear.
Researchers weren't all that satisfied.
Insulin kept in the refrigerator may have been the cause,
all were slightly mystified.

Today, my insulin is back in the refrigerator.
It's no longer an issue.
It is a good thing, for my tears would be endless.
I would always be looking for a tissue.

Within this diabetic school, we consulted dieticians
to learn which foods to eat.
In addition, we were instructed of the utmost importance
to inspect daily our feet.

A doctor, who examined and stressed foot care,
was cracking jokes, trying to be humorous.
At the time, nothing to me was funny,
although he was being polite and courteous.

In observing the room, many patients
    had diabetes due to their obesity.
This was unfathomable, if just losing weight could heal.
    I felt cheated. Why can't that be me?

No physician would have to tell me twice
    to eat correctly or simply to exercise.
Don't they want to avoid the complications
    and perhaps this disease? Can they not visualize?

Perhaps, a nasty virus invaded me
    when I was sick. I don't recall such a date.
I wasn't over the age of forty, not hereditary,
    or from being overweight.

Neither did I fall in the category of pregnant women,
    nor certain ethnic groups.
What actually did happen? Did Fate pull my name
    out of a special hat, making a slight oops?

The mystery has come to an end.
A new life must begin.

After years of unknown symptoms,
    putting me through so much unnecessary agony,
My mom sees it now as ignorance of the medical field,
    friends, and myself, and family.

Of all the doctors I saw, not one noticed
    high sugar concentration in my bloodstream.
It's still today incomprehensible to many,
    since my symptoms weren't mild; they were extreme.

I wish to keep an upbeat mind
   to stay on a healthier and more spiritual path.
In looking ahead for me to grow, evolve, and smile brighter,
   I do need to lose my hatred and wrath.

As a newfound diabetic on insulin,
   I aim to be a relentless fighter.
I need to keep focused on my well-being,
   staying driven to be a healthy survivor.

Others like me are unaware of having diabetes,
   they keep struggling along.
Several have excuses or don't go to the doctors,
   even though they know something is wrong.

There's now more public awareness of symptoms
   and newer drugs for various maladies.
Thanks to advanced media, early detection is easier
   with these newfound remedies.

Chapter III

This has led me to tap further into hidden
    inner resources due to this disease.
I have always and strongly do believe
    that nothing can stop me, not even diabetes.

It has been more than helpful
    to have such an intense inner desire; I can survive.
In just wanting to live a full, active life, be healthy
    and whole, feeling vibrant and alive.

This has led me to tap further into hidden
    inner resources due to this disease.
I have always and strongly do believe
    that nothing can stop me, not even diabetes.

There's no reason why having this chronic illness
    should steal any part of my life or dreams.
I may need to push myself harder to foster
    good emotional well-being to the extremes.

Therefore, I have put myself physically
    and emotionally through many a test,
Rarely leaving myself sufficient leisure time
    for my nonstopping, able body to rest.

This solemn diagnosis interfered with ski instructing,
    so I tried out for ski patrol.
It was a trying challenge, keeping my sugar levels
    under tight diabetic control.

With exerting lots of energy handling toboggans,
    skiing, and giving first-aid,
I kept my pockets filled with nutritious snacks,
    besides having on stand-by an extra band-aid.

On the two ski patrols where I patrolled,
    very few at first knew I had diabetes.
Some were told for my safety due to
    unforgiving trees or other serious injuries.

I wanted to be selected based on my own merit,
    not labeled, or perhaps prejudged.
I am not implying, but being insulin-dependent,
    I made sure I wasn't misjudged.

Before global warming shortened seasons
    and insulin pump, I skied until Mother's Day,
Dealt with unknown energy exertion, keeping supplies warm,
    and shooting up five times a day.

Another challenge was set, questioning
    if I was able to fly overseas again.
Thus, I returned to Europe, revisiting all my
    favorite cities, where I had once been.

Worried about crossing borders, carrying syringes,
    and communicating my needs,
Having low sugars, running out of supplies,
    will I be able to pass by the bakeries?

Reading foreign menus, water unsafe in parts,
    and not easy to find sugar-free pop,
Wine is too sweet and cannot drink beer all day,
    will I be able to keep my body tip-top?

Thus, I plunged ahead and bought an airline ticket
    to roam like a nomad for a whole year,
I stayed six months, not due to my diabetes
    or being surrounded by good German beer.

I had a few problems, but did manage fine.
    I chose later in returning to Europe.
I've learned if I'm focused and have a goal in mind,
    I will not be the first one in giving up.

Even though I was single, I bought a boat
    and I learned how to sail, even sailed alone.
Sailing came easier than managing diabetes,
    thrilling to have bought my very own.

Balancing my sugars was more a worry,
    than heeling over, capsizing was a threat.
I sailed in desolate, distant waters, like Barkley Sound
    and up Princess Louisa Inlet.

The excitement of sailing cheered me on,
    despite the challenging diabetic trials,
Like controlling my ice chest temperatures,
    not warming or freezing my insulin vials.

Being exposed to the elements,
    defrosting a finger for a simple finger stick
And when the boat's rocking and rolling
    in adverse weather conditions, glad I don't get seasick.

Or on a warm, slightly windy day, fearing low sugars,
    wanting to lie in the sun to bask.
An uncomfortable feeling, sailing and diabetes
    are not always an easy task.

My body was kept always in suspense,
    guessing what challenge I was planning to do next.
One summer I dared myself to swim a mile across Case Inlet
    without using a life vest.

Versus the quarter to a half-mile swim
    I routinely enjoyed in the local lap pool.
So, I tested my ability across our cabin waters,
    Puget Sound is chillingly cool.

First, I checked my blood sugar and took the opportunity
    to eat many sweet cheesecakes,
Greased up with Vaseline, like crossing the English Channel,
    convincing two other willing swim mates.

Another friend sailed my boat,
    carrying with him a jug of emergency lemonade.
I had someone else row my dinghy along side of us,
    having it also nearby for aid.

Curious, I immediately checked my blood sugar
    after reaching the other side.
It was so high after exerting so much energy
    and swimming so far; I was shocked and petrified.

Later, found out the cool waters kept my insulin
    from being properly utilized.
Since the swim, I have improved in eating
    more appropriately for when I have exercised.

My next feat was to cycle across
    the Canadian Rockies in 2½ days.
We did some serious pedaling from Cranbrook to Banff.
    I responded in an unreal daze.

I was not feeling well; I had a nasty head cold
    and almost decided not to go.
My bicycle was considered an old lady's bike,
    but did make it, however, I was slow.

I cycled with two competent cyclists,
    who were both supportive and patient with me.
They wouldn't leave me stranded in the wild
    or let me hide if I wanted to behind a tree.

I sacrificed personal things for my diabetic supplies,
    I had to think about weight.
I did carry peanut butter and my sugar-free syrup
    for pancakes for my breakfast plate.

I would make sure to carb up heavily,
    along with eating some protein like eggs or such.
This gave me a weighted feeling for pedaling
    and wondered, if fear caused me to eat too much.

Yet, the worry of too low sugars was outweighed
    by my need to get up each mammoth hill.
I never rode beyond 60 miles before.
    Luckily, I stayed upright, not taking a spill.

Again, distracting myself from all my aches,
    using mind over body, I did succeed.
Getting a Swedish massage in Banff was a great way
    to top off our accomplished victory.

As good as that felt, my sugars can drop,
    so it is hard to relax well and to reflect.
Massages can get my insulin flowing,
    then, fearing a hypoglycemic effect.

Thus, if cycling, I try avoiding my legs for shots,
    I must plan how I will be active.
Therefore, when on shots, I must think twice
    before I shoot up, unless I wish to be inactive.

For a week I floated down the Middle Fork of the Main
    with a boisterous fun-loving group.
We could not turn back once we began heading downstream.
    This was absolutely the only route.

Free from city lights, we were mesmerized
    by the beauty of the luminous galaxy.
Great magnitudes of strength fluctuated with
    each stroke of the paddle, burning lots of energy.

Getting caught in panic moments like escaping sink holes,
    observing my life flashing by,
Anxious on the effects of my unpredictable sugars
    and if we'd lose our food supply.

Others were aware I was insulin-dependent.
    This fact was kept not in secrecy.
I'm glad diabetes or naysayers didn't cause me to miss,
    rafting with such great company.

Nearing 30, neuropathy had advanced,
    so I was sent for an evaluation.
I felt like there's no hope, it goes along
    with diabetes, just another complication.

He instructed, no more electric blankets, wearing nylons,
  or crossing my legs or feet.
As he was explaining to me, I quickly uncrossed my legs.
  He then, pointed to my crossed feet.

I immediately thought, oh no, habits are tough to change,
  can this one habit be beat?
Realizing the importance of what he was saying,
  understanding I must choose not to cheat.

I still get the urge to cross them,
  sitting or lying in bed, but I'm trying to refrain.
For work, I wore nylons less, and if I did, not as long
  since my fears were stronger than my pain.

Running was therapy for me.
  I was again determined to keep putting in my miles.
After this disheartening period, there's been pronounced
  improvements, bringing me many more smiles.

It was a weird sensation not feeling my feet hit,
  just me being jolted as I ran.
Once again, my unyielding tenacity
  kept me running distances, doing the best I can.

After ten ski patrol years, my increasingly impaired vision
  made swooshing down slopes hard.
I was very upset and ready to throw my skis and
  ski boots into a pile to discard.

Lately, I've heard stories of an avid blind skier.
  I needed to hear this earlier.
With the latest technology, he regained his sight.
  Now saying, skiing for him is scarier.

I needed to hear such accomplishing feats
   unheard of to the 20/20 society.
This would inspire, give me hope, and encouragement,
   besides lessening my anxiety.

After shedding extensive tears, knowing,
   snow skiing is a favorite, I bravely tried.
Using low vision tips, I was amazed how well
   I could ski. I was gratefully satisfied.

I was fortunate to have already a strong background.
   I started skiing in sixth grade.
Besides ski patrolling also helped to head
   my skis down most hills without being too afraid.

Knowing the mountain does help and having
   the confidence that I can ski down any hill.
Perhaps, since I'm not an expert, it will not be
   in the best of style or with any great skill.

If I follow a cute gluteus maximus,
   observing reactions of their bodies.
This will alert me to the tougher areas,
   where I might be unable to ski with ease.

I remember skiing close behind, watching
   my girlfriend's white knob on the top of her hat.
It'd bobble up and down, often losing sight of it,
   however, it helped me to ski intact.

If my partner skis too far away from me,
   one needs to wave both ski poles high in the air.
This action matches me with my partner. Since if apart,
   it doesn't help knowing what they wear.

It's embarrassing when I approach strangers
    and act as if it's my husband, Larry.
It's not as funny when I've skied into restricted areas alone.
    That's rather scary.

As a teacher I ran our school's ski club,
    varying up to 90 junior high skiers.
Loads of responsibility, but I managed
    as one of the district's head overseers.

Low vision water skiing was easy except
    knowing when to let go of the tow-line.
The spotter prepared me by waving a beach towel
    as an observable get-ready sign.

This, also, told me I could be more daring and brave,
    crossing more often over the wake.
I'm very pleased to still be able to water ski
    with my friends on wonderful Mason Lake.

Despite my low vision, we owned some powerful
    fast-flying machines, his and hers jet skis.
An adrenalin rush for especially partially blind me,
    as it jumps, splashes, and speeds.

I even had the nerve of opening up the throttles,
    going 60 miles an hour.
The lake was absolutely flat like a mirror
    and vacant of other nautical power.

Most were viewed as unclear craft, so cautiously
    I'd keep my distances by going wider.
Or I would come to a complete stop, beaming,
    I'm not an outsider; I'm a jet-ski rider.

Larry and I powerboated to remote bays in Alaska,
    up the Inside Passage.
Sites where phones, VHF, and compass
    were unable to use, transmit, or receive a message.

Some voiced strongly, "I'd never, ever do that
    and you, with such diabetic brittleness!"
Am I staying ashore, being left behind,
    filling up with unnecessary bitterness?

Of course not, not me, furthermore, my husband and I
    were both fulfilling a childhood dream.
Despite my limitations, my Captain and I, the Admiral,
    make a great nautical team.

Constantly adapting and being reminded
    I don't see as well as I would like to,
I program myself to keep doing my activities
    and be willing to try something new.

In 2004, I learned to play golf with the help
    of my husband's encouragement.
Only being able to see the ball at my feet,
    has not given me much discouragement.

He bought an Odyssey 2-ball putter.
    It helps the sighted to assist me if in need.
I do not always agree, since I don't see the same,
    but I should learn to allow them to lead.

I will continually keep trying to figure out
    some other clever helpful cues.
Since it is difficult to know what tee I'm at,
    where my ball is, or seeing which club to use.

Then, of course, being able to watch and follow
    the path of my husband's or my golf ball.
Some folks cannot imagine and boldly ask me,
    "Why do you even want to play golf at all?"

My goal is not to strive for perfection,
    as I have been too competitive in my past.
I want to have fun, exercise outdoors,
    and meet the challenge, even if I don't learn as fast.

I will do my best not to annoy others
    and to learn some low vision tricks of the sport.
With help from my friends and especially my husband,
    who's my favorite, personal, golf cohort.

After my fourth lesson, I played 18 holes,
    playing far beyond my desired goal.
I was ecstatic by making my first par,
    hitting the ball with surprisingly great control.

The first nine holes were tough, as I was bored,
    lacked concentration, and not having as much fun.
Since I did not detect my subtle, low, 34-blood sugar,
    until I was halfway done.

I do have a streak of stubbornness not to give up
    as this activity is still new.
I'll figure out some diabetic and low vision golf rules,
    and then I'll be ready on cue.

Afterward, feeling great relief, "Did I get my money's worth?"
    I asked my patient golf guide.
"Yes, you certainly played most of the course!"
    was how my witty husband amusingly replied.

Thus, a few feats to see,
  whether or not my disability will stop me.

Hence, if I've made up my mind to do something,
  I'll give it a honest and positive try.
What's there to lose? Maybe a little ego,
  I just don't sit back, allowing myself to cry.

Elated, diabetes doesn't prevent me
  from doing what I like or enjoy.
My spirit may be dampened slightly, yet to feel devalued,
  like an unwanted, useless toy.

I just need to keep my resourceful antennae fined-tuned,
  seeking out creative new ways.
Not all works out, but I can't remain stagnant,
  paralyzing myself for the rest of my days.

The environment and frame of mind of people around me
  plays an influential part.
If negative, limiting, and dragging me down,
  then they're not connecting with an open heart.

I've become aware in how the environment
  can disable you more or can support you.
It was evident while waiting with people
  with varied ailments for a required interview.

I had to show how well I could walk up
  and down steps, dial a phone, and follow a map.
If I'd recognize their transport, and I had to
  walk the block to see if I'd have a mishap.

Enveloped in heavy energy, I felt
   I didn't belong in this distressing scene.
My low vision eyes see myself otherwise.
   I'm not putting myself on the guillotine.

I admit, I do need and want their service,
   however, it was depressing sitting there.
Observing this room of gloom gave me an uneasy feeling
   as I fidgeted in my chair.

All seemed as if lying on his or her deathbed,
   making no visible effort to cope.
Yet, my pump support group, it is upbeat,
   giving me the opposite feeling, giving me hope.

Generally, for the most part, many people will change
   if scared, others will stay frozen.
Fear is one of the bigger motivators
   for the challenging health lessons we have chosen.

It is an ongoing battle with me
   in trying to pass several personal tests,
As I will always be pushing hard, looking for more,
   and trying to do my very best.

Throughout my experiences, I've learned
   by meeting my challenges and facing my fears.
It has given me a feeling of enormous strength
   and empowerment with a lot less tears.

On occasion, my doctor suggested to me to slow down,
   cut back on the exercise.
Nevertheless, being able to do lots,
   my confidence kept positively on the rise.

One of my own beliefs and philosophies is,
    if one wishes to stay healthy and thin.
Then one needs to exercise daily, eat well,
    take nourishing vitamins; use some discipline!

Diabetic material and people remind me
    how complications may occur.
Another reason to resist as I am trying
    to visualize a healthier picture.

During my childhood, my parents have taught me
    good values, character, and to use common sense.
Maybe, at times, I have slipped, however,
    I do go after my goals with lots of confidence.

After conquering feats, I am reassured
    that my life soars despite an unexpected turn.
In achieving goals, I'll eliminate
    any untrue, preconceived diabetic concern.

I'm proud of being thrifty, careful with my finances,
    making more than one sacrifice.
And if need be, working three jobs has all paid off,
    enabling me to do much with a high price.

Most importantly, I've proved to myself,
    diabetes will not stop me, it never will.
I will keep thrusting myself forward,
    even if I can't take a simple diabetic pill.

Chapter IV

One can see why numerous blood tests are essential
and keeping sugar always nearby.
To help maintain balance, I need to keep on testing,
without giving up or questioning why.

After several months of gaining as much knowledge
as I could about diabetes,
My family and I learned a very big lesson,
leaving us all a little uneasy.

When home from college, I was all dressed up,
thinking I was ready for a job interview.
I was feeling poorly, so I laid down,
instead of getting ready, making me overdue.

My dad, Jim, noticed, so he shook me several times,
but I would not respond when talked to.
In a flash, he phoned my mom at work. She urged,
"Call 911!" Both were clueless of what to do.

Jim hoped it might help by gathering up my insulin
and putting it all in a sack.
Nobody was comprehending why I was not moving,
just lying lifeless, flat on my back.

The staff at the hospital came across as most insensitive,
   making me more confused.
As I was becoming conscious I asked, "Where am I?
   What is wrong?" They wouldn't say, they refused.

Instead, the hospital staff would reply by saying to me,
   "We don't know dear, you tell us."
This didn't help. It rattled and panicked me more.
   I'd continue to scream, yell, making a fuss.

I realize it's procedure, checking my mental status,
   seeing what I can recollect.
Yet, they didn't fully understand where I was coming from,
   new to insulin and its effect.

A nurse finally explained I was in the hospital,
   but still unclear why I was there.
My mom could hear me shouting at the top of my lungs.
   This was petrifying, as I was scared.

The nurses kept telling me to be quiet,
   I was waking up the babies on the next floor.
I did not care; I wanted some clearer answers.
   This drove me to continue to fight some more.

As I looked up with unfocused eyes,
   the surrounding faces looked unfamiliar and strange.
It reminded me of the funny farm,
   all slightly altered, distorted, and a bit deranged.

It took such an effort and strain in expressing my needs,
   in getting my slurry words out.
My fighting spirit would not yield or allow them
   to get me to the point of being worn-out.

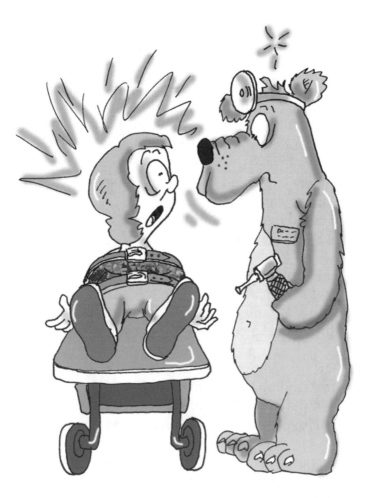

The relentless fight continued for cooperation and answers,
    still so confusing.
Lacking bedside manner, the staff kept giving
    the same impression, that they were refusing.

Then the frustrated staff thought they were being clever
    by strapping down my flailing body.
Being claustrophobic, the situation worsened,
    no one understood, utterly nobody.

They must have not experienced
    such a violent reacting diabetic before.
Or perhaps, they were suspicious it's more illegal drug use
    that is causing such an uproar.

A call was made to my Seattle Endocrinologist,
    he advised, "Bring her in here."
The ambulance also took my worried mom,
    who was permitted to ride with me in the rear.

The attendant showed much more tender-heartedness,
    and was a very understanding guy.
He did his best to explain what was happening to me,
    and said they weren't exactly sure why.

His soft-spoken voice and encouraging words
    were satisfying and good enough for me.
He comforted me by covering me with more warm blankets,
    since I was as cold as could be.

Then the perceptive attendant leaned over,
    turning the oxygen on, as he could tell,
My mom was looking pallid and a little woozy,
    observing, she wasn't doing too well.

With sirens blaring and red lights flashing,
    we rolled down the highway on the most direct route.
I then allowed myself to begin to relax,
    knowing the answers would soon be figured out.

Thus, a terrifying lesson, if your sugars get too low,
    one could become comatose.
Using urine test strips wasn't the best,
    but the main way to keep a close eye on my glucose.

My doctor met and apologized to us
    for going through such an upsetting ordeal.
We just learned another reason why it is important
    in keeping my blood sugars ideal.

My feistiness correlates in how I regain consciousness,
    finding out I want to fight.
If my personality were more meek and mild,
    I, most likely, wouldn't punch, scratch, spit, or bite.

Combativeness can be a sign of hypoglycemia
    and thinking others are mean.
It's my low blood sugar talking.
    I wanted an explanation without the fiery scene.

Keeping my blood sugars near the range of 80-120
    is my ultimate aim.
Yet, as long as I stay brittle,
    above 50, below 200 is now what I'll acclaim.

Mornings best reflect one's glucose level,
    I will celebrate, treasuring if it's normal.
Even if it's brief, my 24-hour goal
    is to keep it from becoming abnormal.

The frequent checking of my blood sugars
　　has become a natural part of my routine.
For security, safety, and comfort,
　　I rely heavily on my blood-testing machine.

Here are more cases with sugar imbalances,
　　understanding they'll never be perfect.
These experiences are teaching others and me,
　　what to do, not do, or what to expect.

Due to being an exception and a brittle diabetic,
　　my life has seen some stress.
I've had my fair share of low blood sugars,
　　putting myself and others through unwanted distress.

My low sugars have created most embarrassing episodes,
　　not wishing to repeat.
Once my boss and a teacher showed up at my home,
　　realizing I was not in my classroom seat.

They watched the medics roll me out,
　　shouting profanity in my least favorite nightgown.
Appreciative, but wished I was invisible
　　to snatch my keys to skid quickly out of town.

I was angry for being so out of control,
　　wanting to run and be an escaper.
Thought it was my turn instead of my students,
　　to receive a happy face on my next paper.

Or when my phone slipped as I tried speed dialing
　　to reach someone to get me some orange juice.
It fell between my mattress and feather bed frame,
　　unable to recover; there was no use.

Hence, I clumsily rolled out of bed, dropping three feet,
    crawling strenuously down the hall.
Not realizing it was still disconnected,
    I tried using the other phone to make my call.

Then dragging myself twice over my vacuum
    to set off my burglar alarm from my den.
Such effort to move my body, to crawl, inching my way;
    when was this nightmare going to end?

Depleted in my ragged nightgown, I'd hope
    I'd be noticed lying across my threshold.
My frightful neighbor misread me as being shot.
    The armed police arrived, acting brave and bold.

It was such an intense mortifying moment,
    lying there with a low blood sugar gaze,
As the police officers raced directly into my backyard
    with their threatening guns raised.

Will they cast me for a crime drama?
    I do not want to wait on my threshold for hire.
If so, to enhance my chances, I need to go shopping
    to buy some new pajama attire.

My low blood sugars cause much frustration,
    and are disturbing when I can't get my point made.
Like when the operator assumes I'm drunk and hangs up,
    unable to convince or persuade.

Feeling helpless and wishing she would do the phoning,
    so I can get some immediate aid.
If the operator only knew how much effort this all takes.
    I'm not a drunk. I'm afraid.

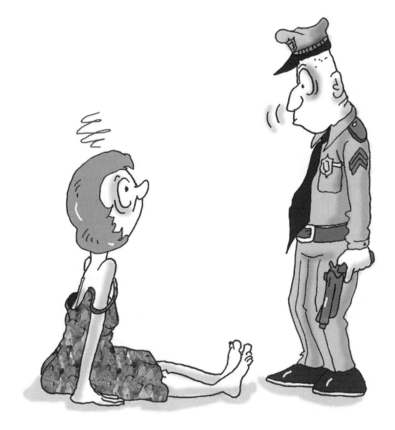

Or the time when my niece wouldn't listen long enough,
   flinging the phone down on me three times.
She was fearing I was an obscene phone caller,
   or one of her friends committing some lewd crimes.

Finally, she handed the phone to her mom,
   who has learned to recognize my slurry voice.
She rushed over to rescue me, putting me at ease.
   I was thankful, now able to rejoice.

Even when I was at a very young age,
   my sister translated what I had to say.
Lucky for me, she hasn't lost her touch
   in grasping the meaning of my gibberish. Hooray!

Serious low blood sugars can be deadly,
   a precursor to a kitchen fire.
It's wise to have others often check in with you.
   It is not what I would prefer or desire.

My dinner was burning on top of the stove,
   luckily, my brother happened to stop by.
I was passed out, lying comatose over my kitchen chair.
   He feared I was going to die.

Jim had previously asked him to check on me,
   dropping in from time to time, if he could.
I was unaware of this and surprised he had;
   yet, felt fortunate, for his timing was good.

He called my dad, and juice or sweets would not help,
   so he was advised to dial 911.
Skip said the medics were admiring my sailboat, flirting,
   and with my burnt meal, having some fun.

Most importantly, they did their magic,
　　bringing my low sugars back to the normal range.
Skip added to my embarrassment by not pulling
　　my sundress down, as it was looking strange.

My brother-in-law always wanted just one time,
　　to break down a door like in the movies.
Since I did not show up at work, they were phoned,
　　concerned it may be due to my diabetes.

My locked-tight house with stout doors was burglarproof,
　　needing to muscle his way through to break in.
He huffed and puffed, breaking both my doors down,
　　hurting his shoulder and bruising his ego and skin.

Not wanting any low sugars while I'm teaching,
　　I frequently checked my blood sugars in class.
My students became educated, learning what's high and low,
　　in this subject they'd all pass.

At first, difficult to grasp that diabetics shouldn't eat sugar,
　　but when low, I did.
They took a genuine interest and assisted if needed
　　in removing my orange juice lid.

My blood sugars can drop to the point of passing out.
　　It's not a comfortable feeling.
It even happened once while I was teaching.
　　This is distressing and not very appealing.

One can see why numerous blood tests are essential,
　　keeping sugar always nearby.
To help maintain balance, I need to keep on testing
　　without giving up or questioning why.

It doesn't always prevent my serious low sugars,
    but certainly does help a lot.
All ten of my sore, poked fingers are rotated.
    I'll keep looking for the next least painful spot.

My very own firefighter is learning what to expect,
    when my blood sugars are incorrect.

Maybe, after the many medic runs,
    the universe at last answered my silent plea,
To have a person with medical training living with me,
    to assist or help when need be.

For the many sleepless nights with low sugar interruptions,
    I did marry the right guy.
He's a Lieutenant from the Seattle Fire Department,
    a gem, who's nicknamed the Cranefly.

He's accustomed to working a variety of aid calls
    on an unscheduled routine,
And ready to take quick action without hesitation
    or the need of a shot of caffeine.

Since living with an insulin-dependent diabetic,
    who does need close attention,
One never knows what to expect, so it's good,
    he's better prepared for unexpected tension.

Once when my good husband was trying to bring
    brittle me back to the state of consciousness.
He saw stars, when I unintentionally decked him,
    almost to the state of unconsciousness.

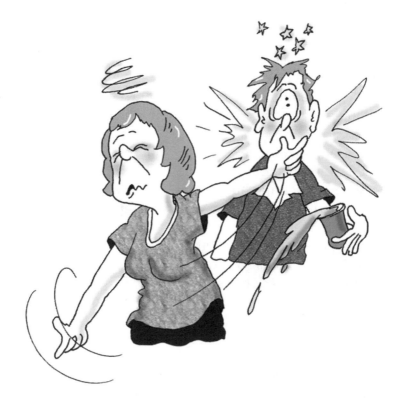

If I can eat or drink when he's trying to raise my sugars,
    he must say, "Chew" or "Swallow."
These words somehow do help me, and I'll do it,
    but he has learned well, knowing what will soon follow.

I will spit out explosively the juice, syrup, or soft candy,
    making a sticky mess.
I'm not trying to be uncooperative
    and put him through more emotional distress.

However, it feels like he is giving me too much,
    feeling like I could possibly choke.
Thus, an unintentional spray comes spurting out,
    getting our bedding, clothes, and both of us soaked.

Here is another example of a late night rescue
    when we both should be fast asleep.
Once again, my caring husband is sleepily aroused
    from him having a deep, peaceful sleep.

He listens to see if it's a diabetic coma
    or my usual chainsaw snore.
He then checks for coolness and clamminess,
    knowing if I am low, I will be cold to the core.

He will next prod and pinch me in sensitive places
    to see if I will wake up or stir.
Then again, he'll listen for a coherent response,
    to hear whether or not my speech will slur.

My husband's worried thoughts are racing.
    Is her glucagon still kept in her nightstand drawer?
He's frantically hoping and wishing I'll wake up,
    saying, "Please, dear, don't bug me any more!"

Then, there are some other bothersome nights;
    I'm wrestling with the covers and our bedspread.
My blurry-eyed husband recognizes another sleepless night
    lies for both of us ahead.

My left foot, both legs, and back are itching.
    It is aggravating. I am ready to scream.
He asks, "Did you happen to forget it?"
    after applying generously anti-itch creme.

"No, not really, maybe for a half a second,
    it is acting like it is here to stay."
I'm praying and imploring for the irritating symptoms
    to rapidly vanish away.

This is just another unpleasant, ongoing battle.
    I guess it is my fated plight.
It's something that's impossible to ignore.
    I'll keep searching for cures; I'll continue to fight.

Dry, itchy skin can go along with having diabetes.
    The itch is driving me nuts.
Caution is needed so my scratching doesn't bleed,
    leading to any possible infected cuts.

When my body is feeling like being overly amorous
    for afternoon delight,
It doesn't really matter what time of day,
    or if it's in the morning, or during the night.

My husband isn't always a lot of fun
    and he can be quick in ruining the mood;
Since his concerns are generally elsewhere at such times,
    not because he is being a prude.

He'll often say to me in a serious, lover-like tone,
    "Check your blood sugar, it is low!"
Then my playmate will know whether or not
    he will be able to let loose and go with the flow.

Yet, hasn't my husband ever realized,
    I just might want to attack him from head to toe,
Even though, my brittle blood sugar is not at the stage
    of being that dangerously low.

Oddly enough, for some reason,
    my low blood sugars do arouse my sexual juices.
In hopes, my hubby has the same passion
    without having any low blood sugar excuses.

For instance, we were out boating,
    after drinking a glass of juice for a low 44.
Charming him with my womanly softness, I whispered,
    "Hey, Captain Dear, come here," hoping to score.

Then using my famous line, "No kiss, no hug, or screw,
    what is a woman to do?" He replied,
"You have a low blood sugar. Does that mean anything?"
    as he turns away, leaving my bedside.

I tenderly murmured in a teasing response,
    "But Dear, I want your body. I want you!"
My Captain responds by admitting, "I would like to, too,
    but the Bilge Rat has things I must do."

Besides, engaging in the joys of sex
    is not as desirable or as much fun,
Let's say for example, if one is experiencing
    a low blood sugar of forty-one.

We both don't always share in sexual pleasures,
    as it can mainly be a one-way street,
Since my body cannot enjoy such activity
    or feel as well from my head to my feet.

My low glucose levels will drop at the most inopportune times.
    It never seems to fail.
Despite what I eat, or my frequent testing,
    it's something I do wish to lessen or curtail.

It does irk both of us, especially my husband,
    who tries hard to refrain from comment.
He understands my extreme sugars, but still gets riled,
    knowing it's challenging, hard to prevent.

When docking our boat or going through the locks,
    I don't want my Captain pulling out his hair.
Therefore, I, Cheryl Lynn, the Admiral of our boat,
    must keep watchful, taking extra good care.

Hence, before docking,
    I must check my blood sugar to see where I stand,
To know whether or not
    Larry will get a conscious helping hand.[1]

Low sugars may be teaching me to slow down.
    It's tough with how fast life seems to have become.
I lead an active, busy lifestyle, but need to smell
    the flowers and listen to the bees hum.

---

1. Excerpt from *Alaska Bound On The Cheryl Lynn, A Mariner's Rhyming Log* by Cheryl Lynn Kantzer Crane, p. 26.

With any low glucose levels occurring,
  my body's great need is to drink some orange juice.
This particular juice will rapidly give me
  the necessary uplifting sugar boost.

I clearly do not fully understand this need,
  why I often keep pushing myself to go.
When my mind and body are functioning at a snail's pace,
  like fighting the sea's strong undertow.

With such blood sugars being precariously low,
  I'm unable to be still and sit.
Even if it is for only a few minutes,
  I cannot stop myself; I just cannot quit.

Somehow, I need to convince myself to wait
  for my sugars to rise as I sip some juice.
My husband knows from previous experiences,
  talking to bullheaded me, there's no use.

As he hollers helplessly, "Stop! Please, sit down;
  wait for your low blood sugar to come around!"
I'm driven to keep pursuing, hearing
  the echoes of his thundering voice in the background.

Then at times, he'll upset me when he blames
  my actions on low sugars and it is not true.
I'll get defensive, however, not violent.
  I do refrain from beating him black and blue.

If I'm excited, talking fast, he'll blame my sugars,
  but it's a personality trait.
Or, if I'm unsure and indecisive when working
  on something I am trying to create.

I am truly thankful for such a doting, loving partner,
    who pays such close attention.
Since my sugars are more recognizable
    when they're extreme, it's difficult for prevention.

Indications of a sugar low,
    they can be subtle and incognito.

The longer one has lived with diabetes,
    the harder the low symptoms are to detect.
I need to be so in tune to reading my body,
    accepting I am not always correct.

It's seldom what I'm logically expecting.
    I must tune in more to my inner voice.
As my callous fingers have realized, it's just another
    simple finger prick, having no choice.

Tingling and numbness around my mouth are
    infrequent symptoms, in which I sometimes can feel.
This feeling clues me in when a low blood sugar is present,
    urging me to eat a quick meal.

Occasionally, I will feel hunger pangs,
    which may be giving me a low sugar sign.
My body is telling me not to waste any time,
    once again, to please go and quickly dine.

Headaches are unnatural for me to have,
    this can be another low sugar symptom.
Therefore, I need to check my sugar level
    before adding food to my digestive system.

One sign as my glucose levels began to rise,
    after being unacceptably low.
Even if the weather is a warm sunny day,
    I'll feel cold as if surrounded by snow.

So, sometimes, I prefer to curl up tightly
    as my whole body can shake, feeling a chill.
My body cannot seem to find the warmth it needs
    as I actually do try to lie still.

Piling blanket after blanket on top of me,
    doesn't necessarily do the trick.
It hasn't taken me too long to discover a sweeter way,
    in which I have found works slick.

I will wrap myself into the warm folds
        of my husband's body, who will share his heat.
Even if we're up skiing in frigid temps,
    he doesn't get cold, including his lucky feet.

I'm not at all bashful in stealing from my personal heater
    whatever warmth I can.
My husband's bare skin knows what's coming first
    as he inhales, preparing for an icy, cold hand.

Thus, I appreciate; I'm able to plug into his warmth,
    nestling close as can be.
He doesn't shy away from my numbing touch.
    He'll lie next to a freezing cold body like me.

Low blood sugars can happen in some uncommon places.
    They can occur most anywhere.
They seem to come and go at awkward times,
    despite knowing what I should do and how to prepare.

When I'm in a crowded public restroom,
    taking extra time for lipstick and to comb my hair,
My nervous husband will send a lady in to see
    if I'm in need with a low sugar stare.

Over the years at home, when my husband feels that
    I've been camping in the bathroom too long.
He'll kindly check on me, intuiting something isn't quite right;
    something could possibly be wrong.

He'll peer suspiciously inside the doorway
    and notice on the toilet there I sit.
Fast asleep, I'm in a coma deep. He's called
    into action, later joking, finding some wit.

When my blood sugars are dropping to the point
    where he can find me in a comatose heap,
My husband will often find some humor by teasing me
    that on the toilet I like to sleep.

He then follows the familiar routine,
    grabbing some sugar to beef my blood sugar up.
He finds my hidden stash of Starburst next to me,
    but prefers using orange juice in a large cup.

He would rather not inject me with Gucagon,
    but will, before he'd call for outside help.
This shot should awaken me in fifteen minutes
    and I won't feel the pain, or give a loud yelp.

When my sugars are abnormally low,
    it gives me this strong feeling I need to pee.
However, there are times when it seems impossible.
    My plumbing won't work, or works too slowly.

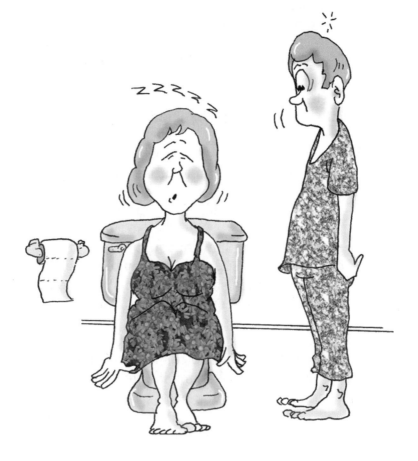

Then, there are moments when I could fall asleep
    if I would allow myself to close my eyes.
Nevertheless, this is how low blood sugars affect me,
    as if they are hiding in disguise.

Therefore, I must prick my finger to self-check
    for my blood's sweetness each time so I can sleep.
This lessens my coma worries and anxieties
    whether I doze off or need to count sheep.

Although it doesn't always seem to work well
    to close my blue eyes for a short power nap,
Since I do not clearly know whether or not
    I am low or tired, feeling honestly zapped.

Thus, it is an insecure feeling, and frustrating,
    when it's not easy for me to know,
In having to deal with such irregularities of sugars
    dropping unconsciously low.

Exercise is a must, a health plus.
    Can it be done without a low sugar fuss?

My mate often teases when out walking,
    how I'll clomp, imitating the sounds of Clydesdales.
It's one of the many signs how my body cries for sugar;
    it's what this style of walk entails.

In addition, my walk can also appear like a drunk,
    slowing to a staggering pace.
While sometimes, I will scrunch my lips into a pucker,
    giving myself a goofy-looking face.

Sweets and change are put purposefully in my pocket,
 ready, prepared, waiting on stand-by.
As well as my blood sugar is checked dutifully,
 before I leave my house, saying good-bye.

It's not surprising before returning, however,
 if I have low levels of glucose.
Thus, I just keep on trudging and pushing along,
 rather than waiting at the nearest fence post.

Moreover, I keep wondering if there's a chance
 for me to possibly lose any weight.
Since before I choose to exercise,
 I surely need to carb up, to up my blood sugar rate.

It is important to walk routinely.
 I actually can slim down, losing some weight.
My energy does increase,
 helping me to feel physically and emotionally great.

My neighbor learned to respect my low blood sugars
 when we were out for a long power walk.
Amidst thick trees, far from the car, he saw that unlike me,
 I was unable to walk and talk.

Having subtle sugar symptoms
 increases the difficulty for me to recognize.
It isn't apparent until they're extremely low,
 or even when it's too far on the rise.

It isn't easy judging how much to eat
 or knowing how many calories I'll burn.
I'm constantly feeling unsure,
 will I be able to stay upright and on my own return?

My concerned neighbor did get me back to the car.
   I was using him as a walking crutch.
He drove me to a drive-in for a sweet drink,
   as my pocket sugar wasn't helping that much.

In controlling and managing my diabetes,
   snow skiing to me is not that new.
How odd it is that I'm fine for a period,
   and then, can be affected the next day or two.

I have learned the hard way that snow skiing,
   soaking in hot tubs, and drinking one glass of wine,
Can be a lethal combo. I must stay alert
   and keep on testing if I choose to combine.

During one fun-filled, long weekend, we headed for
      the ski slopes with fresh fallen powder snow.
We had a dynamite time carving many first powder tracks,
   keeping each other on the go.

We both were eager to return to soak
   our sore, tired muscles in the hotel's hot tub.
Then, our ravenous appetite put us on the food trail
   in search for some satisfying grub.

I struggled and could barely keep awake through dinner,
   or to finish my one glass of wine.
My eyes kept drifting shut, so I suggested,
   "Let's go to bed," I no longer wanted to dine.

Meanwhile, to keep an eye on my health
   throughout the day and the earlier parts of the night,
I had dutifully been checking my glucose levels,
   to reassure myself, they're all right.

In the wee hours of the morning, a slight interruption,
    as time was approaching four.
My husband is sleepily disturbed and is anxious
    in hearing my familiar coma snore.

With my glucagon emergency kit sitting at home,
    he tried his best to bring me to.
Despite his persistent efforts in getting me to respond,
    I would not budge, nor could I chew.

He returned to the same restaurant, hunting
    for some syrup, but it had already closed.
So off to the grocery store he scurried,
    redressing hastily in his warm winter clothes.

The syrup didn't work, nor could he get me aroused,
    starting to panic, thinking, what now?
With my mouth seized shut, noticeable tension
    was hardening his worry lines across his brow.

Called 911 and disappointed, no paramedics,
    they only had an E.M.T.
My husband thought, I'm adept and trained
    as an E.M.T., "Forget it; I'll handle it, just me."

He frantically dressed me in a hurry
    with only my cold weather long underwear.
In the heat of the moment, he didn't care,
    if someone looked at us with a questioning stare.

Using the elevator to get to the lobby,
    he wheeled me down on a luggage cart.
The cart's noise and wobbliness was outweighed
    by his need to transport me, being cleverly smart.

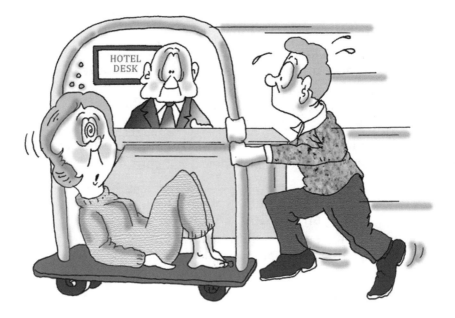

The front deskman's curiosity was piqued
    and intrigued, naturally wondering why.
My able body rescuer explained, asking
    if he would help lift me, "Oh dear me, oh my!"

Our one-ton truck sits high, making it not an easy lift.
    Of course, it must have been a sight.
I guess I was glad, I couldn't feel them lifting my dead weight,
    using their strong almighty might.

Again, through the ice and snow, my sweetheart pulled up
    to the emergency hospital door.
This is not the first time, nor his last.
    He, unfortunately, has experienced this before.

As always, I was grateful my husband,
    who is my personal firefighter, was there,
Since he finds the Emergency workers react too slowly,
    doubting his words like they don't care.

They usually appear, at first, suspicious,
    suspecting an overdosed addict on drugs.
Even after my stressed-out husband explains,
    "She's diabetic, needs sugar!" he'll just get shrugs.

Perhaps, too many previous calls
    due to domestic violence and drug overdose.
Not easy for my medic husband to be a bystander,
    as I'm laying there comatose.

After regaining consciousness, the staff advised me
    to go and get a quick bite to eat.
We slipped stealthily into an all-night restaurant,
    trying to hide, slinking low in my seat.

I was flushed in embarrassment with my husband's parka
    donned over my long underwear.
I still recall getting curious and unwanted stares
    as I was trying hard not to care.

When we returned, walking back through the lobby,
    I could not look comfortably at the guy.
My husband rethanked him; it was now reinforced.
    He wasn't earlier telling a lie.

Who knows what he might have been thinking,
    especially with today's crime, shootings, and violence.
The hotel desk clerk must have believed him,
    since the police were not tipped off, keeping his silence.

I gave my Medic a bad time for dressing me
    with my older, softer, long underwear.
At least I was dressed, but would have preferred
    for the public eye, my other warm, sexier pair.

It's much easier now to snow ski with my pump
    than using multiple insulin shots.
There's no hassle, for instance, digging through
    winter clothing to find some of my exposed skin spots.

With my insulin pump, I still must overload on carbs,
    I was once a normal 93.
I know how carbs turn to energy and then calories,
    but I need many before I ski.

Plus, I set my pump's temporary basal rate,
    decreasing it to seventy per cent.
Yet, after only skiing three runs, I was 78.
    Wow, what energy I must have spent!

I decreased my basal rate to sixty per cent,
    ate an early lunch, stuffing myself more.
I had a large Indian taco with protein, fries, hot chocolate;
    eating can be a chore.

I waddled back out to the ski slopes,
    testing my sugar level after three runs again.
Now a frustrated 70, I snacked on gorp, drank lemonade,
    just plop me in a pigpen.

I was disgusted and riled, so I skied six runs,
    and now, I was a shocking 360.
Was it the cold, altitude of 11,100 feet,
    or was it brittle me?

It's not easy testing in the frigid teens,
    baring my fingers against the elements.
Then, I must squeeze my finger for blood,
    all for better control and preventing ski accidents.

The next day I ate less and put my pump
    at 60 per cent decrease for my basal rate.
I stored juice in my pockets, extra pump supplies, meter,
    and my gorp, in which I often ate.

I ranged between the low nineties, and at the most,
    I had a 180 blood sugar rate.
Each day can be very different skiing,
    and my sugars are not simple to regulate.

I practiced balancing my sugar levels,
    while racing my sailboat, by coming prepared.
It didn't seem to matter what type of foods I ate,
    my glucose dropped, leaving me in despair.

I found the oncoming of dusk, with an added cool breeze,
　may have caused this adverse affect.
Even hot sunshine may drop my glucose,
　weather being the culprit is not what I'd expect.

Furthermore, my husband likes to heat our swimming pool
　to the warm degrees of ninety-five.
Without exerting energy to swim,
　my blood sugars can take a significant nose-dive.

Thus, for my own safety, I make sure there's juice by the pool,
　keeping a close eye on the clock,
Remove my insulin pump, and check my blood sugars twice,
　all in preventing insulin shock.

Once, I almost blacked out in a hotel's spa,
　using snow to cool me down in my panic.
I've now become cautious and less fanatic,
　as spas aren't always relaxing or romantic.

Stress can easily upset my blood sugars,
　as well as be damaging to my body.
Gardening helps to lower my stress load,
　being alone with the dirt, without anybody.

Walking is also one way to de-stress,
　especially after work, keeping me grounded.
I would begin to feel looser and freer,
　and not so physically and mentally bounded.

Both activities can lower my sugar rate,
　I just need to keep eating enough food.
This temporarily irritates and angers me,
　since I'm not always in an eating mood.

I'm a diligent, tireless worker,
    as work is a form of meditation for me.
Especially if I am working in the fresh air outdoors,
    where I don't feel as trapped but free.

If I'm unable to maintain my work level,
    taking notice how my energy has dropped.
My single-focused mind keeps pushing my weakened body.
    My stubborn spirit has not yet stopped.

This is a sign of a low blood sugar.
    I have a tendency to work until I flop.
After reconfirming my unsweetened blood,
    I will then snack, before I'll reluctantly plop.

This has taught me to check my sugars routinely,
    especially if working in my yard.
Sometimes, I'll warily follow a hunch,
    but the subtle symptoms are easy to disregard.

Nevertheless, I will test my sugars hourly.
    They're often unsurprisingly low.
Once, I experimented with Starburst, juice, and nuts,
    taking the time to shell pistachios.

Later, I tried more protein with soda crackers,
    like peanut butter and cheese, besides juice.
Next, I resorted to sugary snacks and candy,
    now having a valid sweet-tooth excuse!

Each hour I would try a variety of foods,
    sweet or not, as my frustration grew.
My stomach stretched, feeling overly satisfied,
    as I began feeling like I could moo.

Sugar results differ with what I eat.
My body dances to its own beat.

Strangely, I can do the same energy tasks,
    and eat the same meals two days in a row.
Senseless, but I'll get opposite blood sugar results.
    It is tiring being a yo-yo.

Two hours after breakfast, my count was 50
    before heading out to walk to keep lean.
I was 190 and had two eggs with two slices of dry toast,
    getting both carbs and protein.

I bolused three point five units of insulin,
    an extra point five for being so high.
Normally, this or three units will work. I can't get riled,
    but must put forth the effort to try.

My 190 reading must have been heading down.
    My glucose machine doesn't give that fact.
And when the same dosage has worked many times,
    I never know how my blood sugars may react.

When I am sometimes in an unhealthy mood,
    for having a caloric and high fat meal,
Pumpkin cream cake and sugar free root beer milkshake,
    in two hours my blood sugar is ideal.

Then, oddly enough, I'll eat Shredded Wheat
    with nonfat milk, and later, chicken lettuce wraps.
My sugar count skyrocketed near 600
    after barely eating merely healthy scraps.

While my pump sometimes malfunctions,
    the cause of this little crisis keeps me questioning why.
I am trying to do my best in controlling my sugars
    from reaching and being sky high.

At 7:00 a.m., I ate one slice of dry toast and
    two grapefruits freshly picked from our own tree.
Then, my blood test at lunch was 316.
    I should not eat a bite. I had to wait until three.

The next morning I ate one grapefruit,
    and ninety minutes later, I was an 83.
This is good. Yet, can I still do my walk, chores,
    and make it until noon with faith and certainty?

It does keep me guessing with my fluctuating sugars;
    I rarely know what to expect.
A grapefruit meal has been eaten numerous times.
    I've even had good blood sugars when I've checked.

There are baffling days when I'll awake
    with a normal 108. My blood's not too sweet.
Then sugars bounce to 363, and for breakfast,
    a cup of fresh, mixed fruit is all I eat.

I'll wonder if my pump's not giving me my bolus
    or my set hourly insulin.
I'll use a syringe to help get it back down
    and subject myself to a prudent discipline.

I'll keep checking my sugars, drink water, not eat,
    and hope my high sugars will disappear.
Until my mystery highs become normalized,
    they interrupt my day and do interfere.

As my day progressed, I'd have low sugars,
  all in the forty range, even a 35.
Every two hours, my mate would keep pinching me
  to see if I was conscious and alive.

It did not seem to matter what I ate,
  and I didn't give additional insulin.
Not until ten did I reach a 158, where my mind eased
  and my sweetheart tucked me in.

One needs to consider such variables,
  like if and how I am being active.
I believe emailing, waiting for repairmen,
  and doing laundry is being inactive.

I wasn't stressed, had no infections,
  medication unchanged, nor did I feel at all sick.
This has been the story of my life; it shall improve.
  A battle I know one day I can lick.

Sugars drop, sugars spike.
  It's unpleasant, not what I like.

For medical procedures for Type I diabetics,
  they are most often scheduled first.
When insulin dependent and can't eat or drink,
  I can't help but worry, fearing the worst.

Not always, but most diabetics can predict and know,
  understanding their bodies best.
It just takes awhile for the medical field to agree with us,
  until they're put to the test.

They can be a tough sell, not knowing or aware
  of my sugars. I'm unsure they'll go well.
First, my early instructions for low sugars failed
  and we could not reach anyone on our cell.

This was before my first colonoscopy;
  I told the nurse my sugars are now normal,
And to please check immediately after the procedure
  as it can become abnormal.

The nurse retorted, "No need to worry, the procedure is short.
  It does not take that long."
After much convincing and repeating myself,
  that afterward, I would still like my blood drawn.

She then scared me by grabbing my pump,
  "You can't have this," thinking it's a pager or cell phone.
I cried out, "You cannot take this, it is my insulin pump,"
  in an upsetting angry tone.

My blood sugars did spike over 300,
  knowing it would not stay in the normal range.
The nurse commented, "Wow, unbelievable, you're right.
  It's shocking they can drastically change."

Moreover, my husband would not leave the waiting room,
  not even for a cup of coffee.
They did not recognize my insulin pump.
  He's not going to leave, he's here protecting me.

Besides, they were unavailable for my low sugar
  as we had earlier discussed.
Plus, having to encourage them to test my sugars,
  explaining they can bounce, how it's a must.

Faith and trust in the Higher forces can be hard,
    knowing things turn out how they're meant to be.
My devoted husband gives me extra confidence
    in trusting he is close and won't leave me.

Besides surgery, other reasons for sugars to spike
    are illness, infections, fevers,
Medications, overeating, any sort of emotional stress,
    like high stressed achievers.

In addition, not having enough insulin,
    or if one happens to eat the wrong food.
All these can cause extreme sugar highs,
    not necessarily putting me in a sweet-like mood.

Sometimes, some or none of the above causes
    climbing sugars, or for me, mine too can drop.
It takes effort not becoming an emergency victim
    or not having my breathing stop.

When high, I'll urinate often, get tired, nauseous,
    and my mouth gets an icky taste.
Before checking my pump, site, or tubing,
    I'll shoot up with a syringe, leaving no time to waste.

When on a sugar high, the more water one drinks
    the better, causing one to urinate.
The body tries to excrete the excess sugar
    through the urine. It is tough to tolerate.

These times remind me of how I felt before my diagnosis,
    which was so horrific.
My high tolerance for pain and discomfort doesn't pay
    when I'm not feeling so terrific.

Hyperglycemia can lead to a harmful condition
    called ketoacidosis.
One needs to check in one's urine for ketones,
    by dipping a test stick to see if one has this.

The body can't convert the blood sugar to energy,
    thus, using the reserve supply, fat.
When fat is broken down and released into the blood,
    it becomes high in acids and that's that.

**Concluding points of my juggling act,
    I'm a fighter; they'll stay intact.**

Neither low nor high glucose levels are good for our bodies,
    both can lead to a coma.
They are serious and can be fatal,
    but it's much better than dealing with a sarcoma.

In my past, while living alone,
    I've lapsed into a coma for longer than a full day.
These serious low insulin reactions are not the picture
    in which I wish to portray.

Medical help should especially be sought
    if high sugars can't be lowered to the norm.
At least, with low ones, your system should produce sugar,
    recovering one's body to top form.

The Hemoglobin A1C shows recent blood sugars
    in a three-month period of time.
This test will show whether the sugar levels have been
    too low, normal, or too high on the climb.

Diabetics should strive for a desired
    target range of 7.0 or below.
Others fall below 6.0, a diet with sweets and carbs.
    For them, there's no need to forgo.

When the results are higher than one is expecting,
    it's a crushing let down if it's more.
Or if the score's great, one's doctor may instruct,
    you are having too many low ones, which is poor.

If I am managing my diabetes with tight control,
    without much leniency,
The sugar level bounces high to low until
    reaching the norm with increasing frequency.

Furthermore, having bouncing blood sugars
    is also not good. It's best to keep them stable.
My aim is to keep my average as low as possible,
    I'm doing what I am able.

My Hemoglobin A1C's are 6.1-6.5.
    It took years to get there.
I'm proud in achieving these low results.
    I've worked hard to improve my diabetic care.

In testing my glucose or shots, blood gets on
    the light switches, clothing, bed sheets, and the floor.
This includes the toilet seat, car seats, counter tops,
    and, of course, in front of my supply drawer.

"Oinketta gets blood everywhere,"
    an endearing nickname by my razzing husband, Larry.
The Blood Phantom leaves undesirable trails,
    if not diabetic, it could be scary.

This is all part of being or living with a diabetic,
     a bloody price to pay.
As much as it bothers me to ruin my clothes, pillows,
     or spendy bedding, what can I say.

I guess one life lesson may be teaching me
     not to strive for flawlessness, as I once did
In dealing with unstable, brittle blood sugars,
     which I didn't have to do as a young kid.

Or is it one of my karmic traits of wanting to take charge
     and be in complete control?
Thus, the universe gives me a chance to deal with sugars
     that are low, high, and rarely neutral.

The bottom line is to take numerous self-stick blood tests,
     to know exactly where I stand.
This self-monitoring of my sugars helps
     in guiding me in selecting the correct plan.

I will continue rotating my ten fingers,
     finding the best one to abuse,
Knowing I really do have a choice.
     However, I am glad it is not choosing to refuse.

Once, a diabetic told me, "I couldn't or wouldn't do
     what you must; I'd rather die."
My sugars may not seem like it,
     but I willingly make an effort and honestly do try.

His remark is ridiculous and depressing.
     His emotions are clouding his vision.
He is destined with this disease, not in managing it.
     His mindset just needs some revision.

Life isn't always predictable like my blood sugars.
    No one gave me a guarantee,
Saying I could sail through life happy, wealthy,
    and free of disease with a healthy warranty.

How do we find our true selves – through religion,
    world traveling, when alone in seclusion?
Or facing life's challenges, the unknown,
    or do we escape into a world of illusion?

I wish to keep both feet planted on this earth plane
    despite the odds and struggles against me.
With life's surprises, like my blood sugars,
    I must think positively on my fated journey.

Chapter V

I constantly need to be resourceful
  in seeking out innovative ways to do things.
I cannot give up and must stay open for suggestions,
  in what society offers and brings.

Another dismal day, my endocrinologist
  noticed spots in the back of my eyes.
He said, "There's no need to worry." My inner voice
  felt otherwise as it turned out to be lies.

Emotionally stunned, fearing two words –
  diabetes and blindness – could I lose my sight?
Pleading, "What can I do?" sitting offensively,
  both of us knowing, if need be, I will fight.

Diabetic retinopathy was beginning to show
  by these emerging red spots.
Sure, we'll keep watching, but how can I not worry,
  upset, with my stomach churning, tied in knots.

Good ophthalmologists checked my eyes on schedule,
  all skilled, specializing in what they do.
The doctors kept moving on to other places,
  as my eye problems continually grew.

My crisp, clear vision worsened to glasses,
    then dimmed to a future not looking so bright.
Now using low vision devices, intuition, guessing,
    as well as other people's sight.

In addition, I'm further developing
    my personal sonar and heightened senses.
Thus, I am discovering new coping skills,
    for a disease with troubling consequences.

Destiny led me to a special ophthalmologist,
    who I like for this doleful plight.
He's supportive, gifted, and found many people
    to help me with my diminishing eyesight.

Many low vision specialists had great ideas.
    I was not as appreciative at first.
Because earlier on, while losing sight,
    I didn't see the beauty of life; I still felt cursed.

For my first laser treatment,
    it took exceptional mind over body for me to lie.
Refraining from comment, I would lie motionless
    for two unwanted needles behind the eye.

I was instructed to lay my arms alongside my body,
    since I was clutching my chest.
I panicked, "Can't do that." "But, you'll hit me."
    I teased, "Not now, maybe later," winning the protest.

After my first laser treatment, my anxiety increased,
    as my eyes were looking grim.
I was forewarned; my night vision would be zapped.
    It'd be harder to see if the lights were dim.

Laser surgery was helpful and did stop some bleeding,
　　but it also took sight away.
From each spot, the doctor must laser.
　　I silently hoped his laser beam didn't go astray.

For my next laser surgery, I strongly expressed,
　　"The pain from one needle is enough.
Please don't deaden the area this time.
　　My high tolerance of pain can handle it. I'm tough."

I was asked if I'd be willing to have
　　my treatment filmed for a commercial for TV.
As long as they didn't film inserting the needle part,
　　that was fine with my doctor and me.

Their intention was to be a reminder for others
　　to have their eyes routinely checked.
The procedure took longer than expected due to filming.
　　I was exhausted and a wreck.

I was infuriated; my eyes were checked.
　　I didn't miss a single eye appointment.
The needed laser treatments were out of my hands.
　　This was such a big, crushing disappointment.

Furthermore, I was a nonsmoker and exercised,
　　maintaining an ideal body weight.
I didn't succumb in balancing my erratic sugars.
　　Plus, I had good blood pressure rate.

After experiencing my two laser treatments,
　　technology had gratefully advanced.
At last, no more needles behind the eye
　　or becalming myself into a hypnotic trance.

This was great news, since I still needed two more.
  I had no control or power to prevent.
My anger was building inside my body.
  I needed somehow a healthy way to vent.

The fear blinded me from seeing anything positive.
  It was in my everyday thoughts.
The simplest things were increasingly harder to do,
  which led to travel and shopping lots.

I had mixed emotions, wanting my vessels to
  stop bleeding, but feared if I'd lose my sight.
My declining eyesight was all up to fate,
  something I, Cheryl Lynn, was unable to fight.

I was scheduled for one of my laser treatments
  to have more surgery on my right eye.
My family had previously bought tickets to see
  the live musical, "The King and I."

It, unfortunately, was showing on the same day.
  I was not in the most cheerful mood.
They thought I should still go; it'd be a distraction,
  but I was being self-absorbed and rude.

Plays are great, but just on the wrong day.
  I was upset, wanting to stay home and be alone.
To close my eyes, losing myself into my dreams,
  and avoiding the rings of my telephone.

Two steps forward, one step back;
  are my planets stressed in my zodiac?

After four laser surgeries, it was helpful
  in stopping my blood vessels from bleeding.
Then much to my dismay, cysts were forming on my retinas.
  We were, sadly, not succeeding.

My ophthalmologist had heard of a specialist
  doing a new laser-type technique.
Technology at that time was limited.
  My situation was unfortunately unique.

Plans were arranged and off I flew
  to meet this retina specialist in San Francisco.
Being out of state, it was a struggle
  for my insurance to agree, a real fiasco.

My dad accompanied me despite his battle with cancer.
  Life was bleak and depressing.
Then fighting to keep my job, driver's license,
  and I feared losing more vision – how oppressing.

At this time, I had other fierce battles to fight.
  Life was filled with so much uncertainty.
I wanted to shield my dad from my own problems,
  like my boss discriminating against me.

When a new procedure and eyes are put together,
  it does not instill much confidence.
Having whirlwind emotions, I was praying
  I'd make good decisions, using some common sense.

My unsettled and rattled being had to look hard
    and search deeply for my hidden smile.
Without the exchange of words, we knew deep in our psyche,
    this eye appointment would be worthwhile.

My options: to be lasered; a risk for instant blindness,
    or it works and my sight does improve.
Or no risk, as my eyes keep deteriorating,
    always questioning did we make the right move?

I am a cautious gambler and usually leaning
    more toward the conservative side.
Yet, my dad and I figured the answer was clear,
    but it was not easy for us to decide.

Much gratitude for my eye doctor's guidance
    in leading me to this gifted specialist.
With his new technique, he treated me three of the four trips.
    Now, thank goodness, there are no more cysts.

This procedure, today, is done by many doctors,
    including now in Washington state.
Timing can be everything, like this opportunity.
    I'm glad I did not procrastinate.

During this same stressful period, my gums were receding.
    I needed to have some gum grafts.
My afflicted transits hitting my natal chart
    were not causing me too many sincere laughs.

Besides seven eye treatments, I had seven gum grafts.
    What is it with the number seven?
There must be a Higher reason, an unclear, hidden message
    being sent to me from heaven.

Many show their caring ways and are kind.
A few can see, but act as if they're blind.

A handicap that is not as easy or as quick to spot,
　　is being legally blind.
Once others find out you can't see as well,
　　a few will not necessarily treat you as kind.

Even if you make it known, trying to explain
　　that you really do not see very well,
There are always a few people, who won't believe you
　　since you appear and look fine, they can't tell.

What symptoms are they expecting to take note?
　　Should both my eyes be droopy down to my throat?
Do I look like a nonsurvivor, sinking in my boat,
　　unable to keep myself afloat?

Many of my conversations will begin by getting
　　confused and slightly misconstrued.
It's difficult to recognize or see whether or not
　　their question is being aimed at you.

I will glance around casually and covertly
　　to see to whom they might be speaking to.
A few people will begin to raise their voice
　　and say directly to me, "I'm talking to you!"

Then, there are a few who'll abruptly change their tune
　　if I keep clarifying and explaining.
I must be patient and have more understanding
　　without getting upset or do much blaming.

Many times, the Sighted, the ones with better vision,
   are the ones who really cannot see.
The example that tops them all was when
   our school's new principal had unjustly harassed me.

I had always received great evaluations
   and took much pride in doing my job well.
I taught, coached, and was ski club advisor,
   and being legally blind, no one could really tell.

Many knew my eyes were changing as I used
   magnifiers, dark pens, and needed large print.
Yet, no one knew, including my close friends,
   that I was legally blind, not even a close hint.

Then, our school hired a new principal and
   she acted as if she was on her high horse.
She had never met me before, nor had she watched me
   perform, yet, she thought she knew best, of course.

Instead, this boss listened to two other teachers
   who were trying to take from me my job.
She summoned me to her office to meet
   and blindly follow their advice; I was being robbed!

The rumors were true; distressed with the added laser
   and retaking my driver's exam.
She told me I'd be unsafe to teach or coach
   and to stay off school property! Wow! What a slam!

Naturally, my family and I were in shock
   and absolutely could not believe.
We were all so puzzled, and they were in doubt,
   so they quickly had to call for themselves to see.

Was this the actual truth? Did I hear right?
　　Could she possibly be saying this to me?
And, yes, other people think she is the one
　　who can see crystal clear? Heaven help society!

Just think of all the low vision and blind folks
　　working competently in sighted careers.
How can she even look at herself in the mirror?
　　Where has she been over the recent years?

In the end, I won the battle in getting my teaching
　　and coaching jobs rightfully back.
She told our faculty she learned her lesson,
　　rumor-listening and impulsive to attack.

Her actions were wrong, so I felt
　　she should have made a personal apology to me.
Instead, she talked in a round about way
　　without any specifics to our whole faculty.

Throughout this entire ordeal, I was instructed
　　to not say or talk to anyone.
As bad news travels, the staff was still clueless
　　of the whole truth of what she had actually done.

Perhaps there is some sort of a life lesson
　　for me in experiencing all of this.
It's how the universe speaks in its various ways,
　　however, without using prejudice.

Realizing some do choose to take much longer
　　adventuring down their spiritual path,
Even though this one has temporarily left me
　　in such a catastrophic aftermath.

Thus, it's crucial in remaining to stand tall,
    keeping myself from biting my upper lip.
As there's a positive for every negative,
    I must learn to handle with a firm grip.

I'm a believer in karma, what goes around comes around;
    she'll get what's coming to her.
One sees daily evidence of this justice, on TV, also,
    that, I'm positively sure.

It's an ongoing battle not letting society
    dwell on my disabilities.
I don't need or want their labels or pity,
    but to focus on my strengths and abilities.

I must keep refueling my drive to accomplish
    and nourish my dreams, accepting my skills.
Negativity can freeze me, lowering my self-worth
    and self-esteem, giving me the chills.

The school incident increased my cautiousness.
    No one should learn of my sight; they'll box me in.
Thus, my visual acuity isn't broadcast,
    fearing more battles I, perhaps, may not win.

Give me time to find my own way in doing things,
    of course, not like those with 20/20.
I've had enough judgments and limitations placed on me.
    The school nightmare alone was plenty.

I am still learning others' accomplishments,
    making legal blindness easier to accept.
The sighted world needs to become aware, too,
    so they can recognize we are not all inept.

An observer may think I have normal vision.
I manage with faith and confidence, lacking indecision.

My eyesight is just for my ophthalmologist
  for knowing how well I actually see.
Having both my eyes impaired due to
  the complication of diabetic retinopathy.

With such profound vision loss, he knows my life
  will be more challenging. It won't be a breeze.
Thus, my eye doctor is amazed in all that I do,
  being in so many activities.

He says I am inspirational, even to him,
  and could inspire other people.
He doesn't know any other patients like me,
  how I am making my life do-able.

He told me his patients with the same vision loss
  do not do a quarter of what I do.
I have no reason to stop now.
  I plan to keep active with my partial 20/20 view.

This explains why when I saw another ophthalmologist
  while vacationing out of state.
He checked my eyes, noted my activities,
  and became curious in how I compensate.

He wasn't as interested in how I saw up close,
  but seeing things at a distance.
I explained, "Really, there is nothing
  except binoculars and my husband for assistance."

The doctor asked me again, "But how do you see?"
    still feeling a bit puzzled and perplexed.
Larry said, "You should have told him that he's the doctor;
    you can still do things, you just can't wear specs."

He rather irritated me at first,
    until my eye doctor kindly reminded me,
Not everyone takes the initiative as I do
    in using the same low vision to see.

My doctor surprised me once, taking me aback,
    as he entered the room before he sat.
I was reading a book using my hand-held magnifier.
    He asked, "Is that how you do that?"

He is not the only person who wonders
    how I get along with my impaired eyesight.
A few individuals will test me to see
    if what I say is actually right.

Once, my curious neighbor divulged, "This may be mean,
    but I was waving at you to see
If you'd notice while gardening. You looked up often,
    but did not see or wave back at me.

I guess you're correct about having poor sight.
    You don't act or look like you can't see that well.
The next time I wish to get your attention,
    I will raise my stern, parenting voice and I'll yell."

I'm legally blind in both of my eyes,
    relying more on my left that's slightly better.
Things take me twice as long as for the Sighted,
    whether it's to read or write a simple letter.

There's a decrease in the sharpness of my vision,
    especially when I'm in the dark.
I don't see specific details, whether male or female,
    or facial features, like a birthmark.

I can see large shapes, but not crystal clear;
    I do get privately envious.
My peripheral vision was not as affected,
    so I'll twist and turn my head to focus.

My husband gets uneasy if I direct him
    to drive to a friend's house for him to meet.
Because, unlike me, he likes using street signs,
    addresses shown on the houses and on the street.

Context, size, colors, and general configurations
    help me identify a word.
Sometimes, it's that wide-spreading tree or ten-foot fence.
    It's never the little street sign that's named 'Third'.

My low visual aids keep me informed, helping me to see.
    They are beneficial in keeping my life stress-free.

Too bad impaired vision devices are so expensive.
    They can make life less burdensome.
Some aren't as powerful or available when needed,
    but keep tension to a minimum.

My CCTV from Division of Blind Services
    was for teaching, a useful tool.
It took awhile to get use to it, but once mastered,
    I loved it, leaving it mostly at school.

This CCTV looked like a TV screen.
It sat on a rolling electrical cart.
It would blow up the print, shown in black on white
or the reverse, could write or draw, doing some art.

It was cumbersome, large, and inconvenient
to bring home daily or for vacation.
Nevertheless, I transported it each way if I needed it.
It was worth the frustration.

Even a few of my low vision students would use it,
making their lives easier, too.
Again, why must these devices be costly
and easy to buy for mainly the well-to-do?

My CCTV is now too old and in dire need
of some major costly repair.
I'll need to shop and explore newer models,
taking time, energy, and money to compare.

Each day, teaching was an enormous challenge,
but I was proud of what I did achieve.
I read 90% of our classroom books
to help encourage my nonreaders to believe.

The onset of the school year was taxing and wearing,
learning student names with their faces.
Taking attendance and keeping my gradebook neat,
lining up and putting grades in tiny spaces.

I can't read what I write unless it's written very large,
too large for correcting papers.
Meanwhile, I keep close tabs on my blood sugars,
so I'm not teaching with any low sugar slurs.

I do appreciate my CCTV, magnifiers,
  and magnifying glasses.
I get annoyed untangling my glasses' cords,
  or with my jewelry, or cords of my sunglasses.

I relied on an extra-large seating chart
  written with a bold black permanent ink pen.
Quickly tuned into their voices
  and ran a tightly organized classroom regimen.

Kids often wore the same jacket or clothes
  with their own individual style of walk.
It was also impossible in seeing
  the minutes on my extra-large numeral clock.

Correcting over 600 weekly papers
  with their various styles of handwriting,
Even requiring typed, black, or dark blue ink,
  still made it hard and I needed more lighting.

The Services for the Blind helped somewhat
  by attaching to my desk a fluorescent light.
It aided me when my classes watched movies,
  or whenever my room's lighting wasn't as bright.

With lights or not, running audio-visual equipment
  was tough unless memorized.
Furthermore, computers weren't set up well
  for my impaired eyes as school became computerized.

Thus, helping students with computers,
  or using the school's or public library.
Or the ease of reading just a page number
  without using an aid that was necessary.

As exhausting as all this may seem,
  I did enjoy teaching, especially for junior high.
I took frequent mental and physical retreats,
  willing to ask for help, and couldn't be shy.

I was aware it was not in my best interest
  to be pessimistic, sulk, or pout.
Be that as it may, there were some tiring days.
  My patience was worn thin, and I was worn out.

My mom had inquired, finding a beneficial plan.
  She was being ever so sweet.
Understanding me well, she knew to conquer losing sight,
  would be an enormous, trying feat.

Twenty years ago my parents treated me
  to a low-vision conference in Denver.
It left a favorable, lasting impression;
  I will not forget. I'll always remember.

It really opened my low-vision eyes further,
  altering my narrow mind-set much more.
Becoming keenly aware that my life is certainly not over,
  nor need it be a bore.

As I learned many present and new developing
  low vision and diabetic tools,
It felt to me as if I was returning to one of the
  more meaningful, life changing schools.

It was also incredibly impressive to watch
  how blind people were able to scoop,
After nature did its calling, picking up with their baggies
  their well-trained seeing-eye dog's poop.

One favorite product I enjoy recommending
    for helping others become aware,
Are the DVS movies that are intended mainly
    for the blind and vision impaired.

This is a descriptive video service,
    describing movies between the dialogue.
It gives us a lot more detail of what's happening,
    instead of leaving the blind in the fog.

Even those with 20/20 take pleasure viewing these movies,
    they don't seem to complain.
Once, my spouse saw a few details he had missed,
    like when they were describing parts of an airplane.

Today, my mate will DVS TV for me.
    I certainly can and do miss a lot.
With quick action or actors looking too similar,
    I have trouble in following the plot.

It helps to use varying shapes or sizes of magnifiers,
    either with lights or not.
All have nearly the same magnification.
    A few are placed purposely in a special spot.

Like for kitchen use on top of our microwave,
    there is a small, unlighted one in size.
They are spread strategically throughout our entire home
    for my impaired low-vision eyes.

The stronger the power, the smaller the magnifier;
    it's too bad it's not the reverse.
I suppose looking at it with positive eyes,
    it's easier to carry within my purse.

A magnifier with a halogen lightbulb is the brightest;
    keeps me from less guessing.
At times, it will take awhile to read one little word.
    I can't allow it to be oppressing.

One sunny day, sitting on our sundeck,
    I was reading our mail with my magnifier.
I took a water break and smelled something burning,
    but thought who would be now having a fire.

Although it smelled quite close and pungent,
    I scanned our neighborhood and tried to follow my nose.
Then shocked, it was my reading materials smoldering.
    Relieved, there was no need for our hose.

This now explains the many scorched spots
    on my papers, or scorched fabric on our furniture.
I'll cover these reading tools so I don't leave
    my unintentional arsonist signature!

Plus, when reading in the sunshine
    with magnifying glasses as my low-vision aid,
My eyes have a tendency to dry out,
    even if I am wearing my sun visor for shade.

Large print books are great, but for me, the print is
    still disappointedly not quite the right size.
They're heavy and awkward for using magnifiers
    or my glasses, holding the book close to my eyes.

With large or small print books, my hand gets tired,
    holding my magnifier up in the air.
It'll fall asleep, so I must keep shaking it.
    It gets annoying, but it's one thing I must bear.

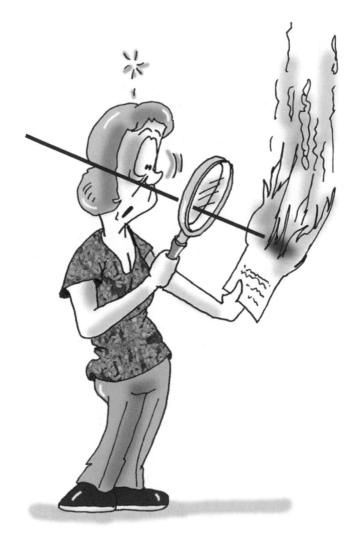

Glucose test strips that pull the blood over
    are the easiest to use with impaired vision.
They enable me to test my own glucose levels
    without any help or supervision.

For testing my sugar level, I obtain blood
    from the side of a well-used fingertip.
Then I will hold the strip's edge near the drop,
    waiting as blood moves magically onto the strip.

I love using my talking computer program
    with its contrasting, large-printed keyboard.
It'll enlarge the print on the screen; however,
    the frequent updates get expensive to afford.

It reads aloud as I type along, relying more
    on my ears for correcting a mistake.
Or, if I wish it to read a document,
    I'll sit back and listen, taking a typing break.

This computer program for the visually impaired
    has more features than I am aware.
I can use email, internet, word processing,
    and communicate with others everywhere.

I have this profound ability to concentrate,
    losing time and forgetting to eat.
My mate says, "You have an astonishing ability
    to turn to mush," raising his heartbeat.

Since it's too easy to remove myself,
    drifting away from my surroundings mentally,
It's most helpful in using the hourly alarm
    on my talking watch in reminding me.

My watch has four other alarms with verbal greetings.
    Besides the time, it gives the day's date.
It has a stopwatch and can be set by using my ears;
    for my low vision it is first-rate.

I get a variety of remarks when using
    my talking watch around other folks.
Most, not fully understanding why, would say, "Wow!
    Where'd you get that?" while others tease, cracking jokes.

A most unusual comment when someone heard
    my well-used little talking time machine:
He said, "Oh, you're one of those. You can't tell time.
    You must be from California." What's that mean?

For walking, my neighbor thoughtfully gave me
    a worthwhile gift, a talking pedometer.
It measures distance, time, calories, steps,
    and if I divide, it becomes a speedometer.

I did not know such a thing existed,
    what a truly practical low vision device.
Perhaps hearing calories burned may help balance me;
    the information seems to be precise.

I'll keep finding various useful tools.
    I won't refuse the help of a low vision store,
Or from my friends, family, catalogues, conferences,
    and other avenues to explore.

I want to stay as close to the sighted world as I can.
Safety is a concern, but staying active is my plan.

I can't always wait for others to help.
   Ideally, I'd like a full-time secretary.
More than once, I must do what I can,
   whether or not for the low vision it's customary.

Our hotpad on our boat fell apart.
   It would no longer hang, so it needed to be sewed.
I commanded my Captain, "Please, thread the needle, I'll fix it."
   Grinning, he quickly replied, "Oh, no!"

I've never even come close in being a seamstress,
   nor can I see specific detail.
Yet, I was more than willing to try to sew it.
   It's just a hotpad, who cares if one can tell.

However, my sweetheart was more than willing to assist.
   He donned his helping, tailor hat.
Knowing it is a lot less taxing on him,
   but I would enjoy the challenge to have sewn that.

My Captain and I do have tense moments out boating,
   where we get riled with one another.
Being as active, my vision loss escapes his memory,
   or sometimes, he tries to smother.

Once, for a brief moment, *I had to steer,*
   could not keep on course.
Partially due to fog and now finding out
   using only one engine force.

Captain, unhappy with me, told me
  'Don't ask me to steer;
I don't want the job.
  You can do it all from here.'

I had made an unknowing
  180-degree turn,
I guess unconsciously
  I wanted to return.

He forgets, I must look through binoculars
  to watch out for debris.
Meanwhile, to look at instruments that
  I can't really see.

Even if it's not foggy,
  to find an object to help direct me,
He's clueless; steering for me is not a breeze,
  'Please, let me flee,'

He needs to start investigating
  for more low vision gear.
That could make it a lot easier
  for me to steer.

What did the blind man
  who sailed to Hawaii use?
Need to find out
  so I am no longer verbally abused![1]

---

1. Excerpt from *Alaska Bound On The Cheryl Lynn, A Mariner's Rhyming Log* by Cheryl Lynn Kantzer Crane, p. 72

One time when we were ready to gather our shrimp,
    Larry hurt his back on the first shrimp pull;
Began to get nastier
    than a raging bull,

I suggested
    in switching our two roles.
He hesitantly steered.
    I grabbed the pole.

I luckily hooked
    the first pot fine,
With the Captain
    nervously standing behind.

He yells, 'You can't see it,
    Let me do that.'
I shouted in return,
    'No, I'll do by best. Scat!'

With much luck,
    we did get both pots in.
Yet, it was not easy keeping Larry
    where he should have been."[2]

Therefore, I am still processing, just because
    one does not see as well as one would like to.
It does not mean to me one needs to stop living,
    or that one should allow others to stop you.

---

2. Ibid, p. 117

My intentions are not to cause my husband's blood pressure
    to rise with too many upsets.
I only want to have the opportunity to try
    without giving him any regrets.

I can be a klutz, making low vision mistakes.
I now can laugh until my body aches.

The sighted and vision-impaired have done this,
    as partially blind bat me has done this, too.
Some, unconsciously, have entered the wrong restroom.
    I luckily withdrew once I had a clue

Unlike my sister, she and a friend made it as far
    to sit on the pot in the men's room.
They noticed the shoes in the next stall were not female,
    but male, feeling an impounding, dark doom.

They sat frozen in awkward embarrassment,
    glued to the toilet seat, unwilling to budge.
They stayed hidden until all was clear, then scrambled
    before any upsets or they'd be misjudged.

Situations like these need to be remembered,
    but really, how could one ever forget?
It shows when my sight causes me to do things.
    It's not as bad as I think; there's no need to fret.

My vigilant, on-guard mate says,
    "You need to stand at attention before leaving the house."
He'll often catch me if I'm dressed inappropriately;
    thank goodness for my seeing-eye spouse.

He's not foolproof. Once standing in front of my class,
    immersed and focused on my instructing,
I felt my feet were swimming loosely in my shoes.
    Then, a roar of laughter began erupting.

As I screeched, "Oh no, I have my husband's tennis shoes on,"
    the students laughed along with me.
My lesson came to an abrupt stop.
    With the out-of-control laugher, I fell down on one knee.

At the end of school, I'd have my students
    list twenty things they remember about their year.
Naturally, nothing intellectual was listed,
    but can you guess one popular thing you'd hear?

One day, I was sitting on the edge of our pool,
    my husband points out with a smirking frown;
I don't know how, but I was wearing my swimsuit inside out
    with my swim goggles upside down.

Once, after rushing home from a luncheon,
    I threw on my loose-fitting shorts and a tee shirt.
I took a home computer lesson. Then Larry returns
    and chuckles, asking if I'm alert.

I was wearing my shorts inside out and backward –
    wow, I cannot believe. How did I miss?
Goodness, gracious me, this is so embarrassing.
    Did my instructor happen to notice this?

My husband teasingly adds, "It's good I know you.
    I could be given the wrong impression
and flown into a jealous rage with suspicion,
    filling with unnecessary aggression."

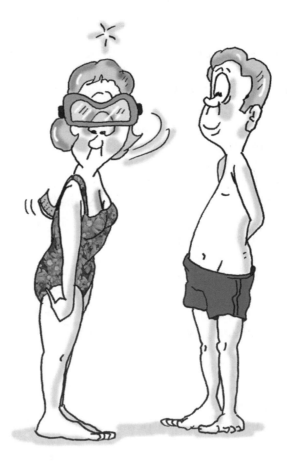

No one has said I was perfect, though I might like
to lead others to believe I am, HA!
Do I have to admit to myself that
I might possibly have just one tiny minute flaw?

However, once showering, Larry bursts into laughter,
pointing down to the shower floor.
I had unknowingly stepped in with my slippers,
but what's new, I've also worn them to the store.

It's healthy having many hearty belly laughs,
as it can be amusing in our house.
Since life can be too serious and depressing,
I'm lucky living with a good-natured spouse.

There absolutely needs to be a healthy balance
between seriousness and lightness.
Without having humor, our life can look dim.
We need daily doses of sunshiny brightness.

Our emotions can cloud our vision.
Therefore, I'm learning to forget, forgive, and release.
I've had to make deep changes within myself,
so the negativity and bleakness can cease.

When I wash dishes, my driers keep a sharp lookout,
making an eagle-eye inspection.
They are worried about bacteria being missed,
leading to illness or an infection.

No matter how many times my drier returns
the dirty dishes back to me for rewashing.
I do not let the rejects bother me.
I now can handle more jokes and a lot more joshing.

Therefore, when the rejects are returned,
    after they're washed, rinsed, almost dried, and still are icky,
My drier jests with me, "Are you planning to leave this sauce?"
    I'll tease, "You are being too picky."

For work, I will purposefully wear two different earrings.
    My kind students will point it out.
Like, I've worn a sailor on one ear, and on the other,
    a sailboat prepared to come about.

In this way, I am appreciative of the support
    and all the assistance I can get.
I will not turn down a helping hand from family,
    friends, students, or even strangers I've met.

We are more alike than some want to admit or believe.
    Our lives twist and turn, challenging us to achieve.

Like my former boss, there are those people
    who don't seem to see with 20/20 vision.
Some forget, are clueless, or see too narrowly,
    where their thought processes need some revision.

Our similarities to one another,
    is a concept that's not easily embraced.
When one has a disability, she's labeled
    and our commonalities are all erased.

Thus, the Sighted can be difficult at times,
    in needing a wake-up call with a good smack.
I need to maintain self-control. It's better than taking revenge
    and going on the attack.

Like asking Captain Larry to refresh me
    with changing the channels on our VHF.
"I've showed you how to do this many times before!"
    he impatiently yells, as if I am deaf.

He will show me with agitated, exaggerated actions,
    but his wrath is ignored.
Because I've learned his eruptive tantrums don't last long;
    knowing his sweetness will soon be restored.

It's true, he forgets I don't see and must memorize it.
    I haven't done it for a year.
So as each boating season approaches,
    I must be reacquainted with our nautical gear.

One learning style for me is the more I physically do it,
    the easier it'll get.
Whether I see well or not in what I'm doing,
    if repeated, it helps me not to forget.

One time, my 20/20 sighted husband was frustrated
    while dialing our cell phone.
His erratic fingers kept misdialing
    when trying to retrieve our messages from home.

I must remind him on occasion,
    as I chuckle at his "sighted-disability."
This should aid him in giving me much more compassion
    when commenting on my utility.

Even my strongest low-vision devices
    do not enable me to read some small print.
Fortunately, for me, my good hubby is there,
    but for him, patience would be a helpful hint.

Once a steward joked, "Are you sure you can read that?
    You're reading so close," brushing my elbow.
I responded, "These are magnifying glasses. I need to..."
    as he chuckles on by my row.

Some inquire, or tease, or make inappropriate comments
    wanting an explanation.
I don't mind clarifying, solving the mystery;
    I object to inconsideration.

Especially when we complain about others,
    we need to take a closer look at ourselves,
Since it can be our shadow or dark side
    that is being mirrored at us, our true inner selves.

I, also, can get increasingly frustrated to the point
    where my clear thoughts won't come through.
I'm still learning to sit back and relax completely,
    so I'm able to plan what next to do.

I constantly need to be resourceful
    in seeking out innovative ways to do things.
I cannot give up and must stay open for suggestions
    in what society offers and brings.

I am partially at my wits end and dissatisfied
    when I'm dependent on someone.
Yet, independent I must realize, I, too, can help others,
    including my sweet honey bun.

The person I'm evolving to be,
  does feel lucky in how well I see.

Some people do not wish to take the time to read,
  they're motivationally deficient.
And, sadly, there are some who are illiterate and incapable,
  nor are they proficient.

Then there's a breed who shouldn't work for the public.
  They get annoyed and their sun does not shine,
If asked to read the menu, a posted sign,
  or to identify food in a buffet line.

Even after giving them my rehearsed line
  of not seeing well, I only see somewhat.
Some serving the public disappoint and should be pleasant
  and helpful, whether one sees or not.

Despite the quizzical looks, there are those
  who are truly wonderful and most generous.
Thus, it's a waste of time and energy
  to get my ire up, becoming too furious.

Maybe some would be more understanding, sensitive,
  and without hesitation be kind,
If I'd accept the cane offer from the Lions Club,
  andgive up skiing, to wear a sign I'm blind.

I, honestly, would not hesitate if it's necessary,
  or I'd greatly benefit.
I've learned my stubbornness doesn't pay in all things.
  In this lifetime, I'm not a total nitwit.

With great emphasis and deep conviction,
　　we are who we are, whether we like it or not.
And my husband and I are happy to say,
　　I'm doing fine. We'll continue smiling a lot.

Some are confused and ask why I don't wear glasses.
　　This concept is often misunderstood.
I guess since I appear so "normal" to them.
　　I certainly wouldn't hesitate if I could.

My fate is my magnifying glasses
　　and the other low-vision devices I use.
I can't believe when glasses did help me, I was so vain.
　　They were not worn much. I did refuse.

Now I'll wear my unattractive thick-rimmed glasses to read,
　　if I'm out in the public eye.
I'm unconcerned with them not looking so slick,
　　or trying to hide in a disguise, being shy.

In teaching, I explained, "Yes, these are ugly.
　　I feel like an old lady. But for me to read,
I will do what it takes, whatever I will need,
　　even if it's not up to my fastest speed."

I hope I made a powerful impact,
　　mainly for my Remedial Reading students,
By witnessing my effort to read the board, books,
　　schoolwork, or educational documents.

I felt like a true kindred spirit, as I too
　　have to persevere to struggle to read.
It is just in a different fashion, as I wondered
　　if they realized I had the same need.

If one identifies with similar problems,
    it's possible to teach and heal someone.
I would be delighted if only one student connected
    and could make the comparison.

It's ironic, I have my Masters in Reading,
    and Reading Resource Specialist degree.
Yet I can't see well enough to read print in books.
    Was this a Higher plan of how I would be?

A half-blind friend said it's imperative
    to keep physically and mentally active.
We agree it helps from dwelling on the negative.
    Many vision-impaired are inactive.

To help keep my mental faculties stimulated,
    I've fallen into a new routine.
I enjoy the mental, not physical challenge,
    of doing a crossword puzzle magazine.

I juggle with magnifier and glasses to read,
    write in, or use the dictionary.
I do what is necessary, as it also
    expands my limited vocabulary.

My glasses are not always quite strong enough
    to read the clues or the numbers correctly.
If I just can't figure one out, I'll ask to double check.
    I often see it incorrectly.

The large print puzzles aren't as interesting
    and are still hard to see a number or clue.
Some shapes are easier to read so I'll read
    forward and backward to find one is what I do.

But it does take magnifying glasses and
    my magnifier to fill in one small square.
I will do what I must and will put up with such fuss,
    the lucky sighted are just unaware.

Thus, many people do take their eyesight for granted,
    as I also did some years ago.
It is a reminder to take that extra step
    without feeling sorry for my story of woe.

Sometimes, I forget how well I see, or rather not see,
    as I shop at the same local store.
The store went through a major remodeling.
    This was unsettling, clear to my inner core.

I'll save many steps if I keep shopping at a store,
    until its aisles become familiar.
It's tough comparing costs, analyzing nutrition facts,
    and products look all too similar.

Yes, I do miss the comfort of reading anything
    and anywhere without assistance.
I'm envious watching others wearing sunglasses
    with their material at a distance.

If they do not have to deal with major vision loss,
    it'll be something else they'll have to face.
So my visual impairment isn't so bad after all,
    I am in a much better place.

It is an inescapable reminder each day
    in how much my vision is impaired.
Yet my mind focuses differently at times,
    causing me frequently to be unprepared.

My mate and I attended a talk,
 forgetting my magnifier at the restaurant.
I convinced him. I'll run back alone to fetch it.
 I knew this area; I was confident.

It was getting late, as darkness was rolling in
 and dusk was just about to disappear.
We were only a few minutes away, not that far.
 We'd been here numerous times this last year.

All I could see were many bright lights,
 unable in distinguishing the restaurant's light.
For a panic moment, I realized I really don't see that well,
 questioning which way was right.

I heard a clerk locking her store. I shouted, "Which way?"
 "There," she pointed in the direction.
I yelled, "Can't see well, am I pointing right?"
 "Yes, across the lot near that busy intersection."

Brief moments like this bring me back to reality,
 reminding me I don't see as well.
Thus, it's good my mind sees it positively,
 telling me I'm capable and can still excel.

Limits and boundaries do need to be recognized,
 while keeping a positive outlook.
This is one of the main reasons why it has guided me
 to the very writing of this book.

Both my right and left eye have been thankfully dry
 and stable for the last several years.
This news of good health brings my family, friends,
 my doctor, and me to yell with many good cheers!

I'm glad being legally blind doesn't stop
  Larry or me from having such fun.
We both know that our good life is not over,
  and we're definitely not done.

We always have a good story
  or two to tell,
'What, all lies

  in your very own wishing well?'[3]

3. excerpt from *Alaska Bound On The Cheryl Lynn, A Mariner's Rhyming Log* by Cheryl Lynn Kantzer Crane, p. 58.

Chapter VI

Low vision has been teaching me to use my six senses.
    This also includes my third eye.
Many folks are still unaware or do not wish to accept,
    and sadly, they choose to deny.

My goal is to gain more knowledge in keeping
    my blood sugars in a balanced condition.
Due to subtle symptoms, I rely on general feelings,
    analyzing my activity, blood tests, and my intuition.

Recognizing our psychic abilities means
    one has a sense of direct knowing.
When we forgo our conscious use of reasoning,
    we'll continue to evolve and keep growing.

People who think intuitively act instinctively,
    having absolutely no doubt.
We all have the innate ability to be intuitive,
    but we've learned to block it out.

Or, we rely too heavily on others,
    mainly those holding prominent positions.
The ultimate choice is ours, but we allow them
    to influence our personal decisions.

Most are authorities who mean well with good intentions.
    We need to respect their advice.
Yet, it is important to listen to our first instincts,
    without the need of hearing it twice.

Whether or not it is our medical professionals
    who help manage our health problems,
We gladly listen, in hopes to eliminate our concerns,
    marking off our poor health items.

The more we value or trust our inner selves,
    the more our own intuition will blossom,
Leading us to reach new dimensions or universes
    unknown to us that are quite awesome.

The ultimate inner guidance comes from inside,
    the importance is to have faith and trust.
The more we trust our intuition, the more we trust ourselves;
    it isn't easy to adjust.

With low vision, we're forced to rely on
    using other senses for our survival.
Or, our sixth sense which has an unexplainable
    and mysterious way of arrival.

As one's inborn latent talents are expanded
    and slowly begin to be uncovered,
Who knows what awaits us – what practical,
    well-needed survival skills will soon be discovered.

I've had to open and explore my psychic sixth sense,
    which lies dormant within most of us.
It's just an unconventional way to help get around,
    an added plus with a lot less fuss.

There's still room for me to improve,
  slipping into the astral world groove.

I'm still learning how to use my intuition
  and to listen to my inner voice.
If I had it down 100%, my life would be easier;
  I'd openly rejoice.

I always will, and presently, I'm still realizing,
  that I have plenty more work to do.
Here is a small, colorful example of how
  I picked up a pile of some nasty dog poo.

As I was admiring our impeccable, green lawn,
  I reached for some in our front yard.
I had mistaken it for an unwanted fallen leaf
  that disturbed me; I wanted to discard.

My sniffer wasn't working, but my touch sense
  led me to this disgusting discovery.
Times like this I'm learning to laugh
  to keep myself on a positive road to recovery.

Another example: I once began to remove
  a live floating bee from our swimming pool.
Until my sister with her sharpened eyes shouted,
  "No, that's a live bee, that wouldn't be too cool!"

I had caught a glimpse of something dark
  floating in the water, thinking it didn't belong.
Even though my inner voice shrieked, "No, it's not a leaf,"
  I still reached out, not knowing it was wrong.

In dining out, I accidentally ate my lemon wedge,
    which I had used for dressing.
Spitting it out in an embarrassing gag reflex,
    my manners at times are not impressing.

This time my brain's logical side wasn't working too well.
    It wasn't its first time to fail,
Being that I had just finished squirting my salad,
    leaving a low calorie lemon trail.

In Arizona, I was getting ready to do laundry
    in my mom's washing machine.
I first peeked inside and immediately noticed
    how her machine did not look so clean.

Gingerly, I reached inside to pick up the unknown
    dark substance to see what it might be.
Unable to see the specific details, my next thought was,
    maybe, I should first ask Larry.

Feeling the pounding rush to drop it quickly,
    I was urgently calling for him to see.
My husband shouted, screeching in shuddering disgust,
    "A DEAD SCORPION! Oh, dear me, dear me!"

Therefore, as one can clearly see, more work lies ahead,
    although much improvement has been made.
I must keep on stretching my learning as much as I can,
    in finding whatever gives me aid.

Do we have a clue
to what our bodies can do?

Our bodies keep receiving messages
    and probably often think we're not so bright.
Since we're not heeding the signs, yet, the universe knows,
    some day, we will hopefully get it right.

I am personally wishing to learn
    how to heal myself from my diabetes plight.
This will also develop my third eye much further,
    and will enhance the use of my eyesight.

The voices coming from our bodies should not be ignored.
    They do need to be listened to.
These strong messages will not be misguiding.
    They're uncanny, accurate, concise, and true.

We need to be profoundly more appreciative
    of all the things our bodies can do,
As well as the little disregarded minor things
    that we easily take for granted, too.

We often criticize, rank, and make fun of our bodies,
    or we will overdo too much.
We'll push until we can't use a finger, have a sore foot or back,
    our elbow won't bend, or such.

We service our cars, furnaces, and some machinery
    to run at peak efficiency.
Yet, our bodies are irreplaceable and need fine-tuning.
    We don't have that same tendency.

What kind of messages are we giving our body
    from keeping it healthy, strong, and sound?
Consequently, we must hear that familiar tune,
    that wise saying, what goes around, comes around.

*Should our visual acuity
    include our psychic intuity?*

Since one sense is weak, others have become stronger,
    further developing my third eye more.
It certainly has awakened my low-vision eyes,
    opening up an enlightening door.

I'm in the process of fine-tuning my other senses
    to make up for the loss of sight.
Realizing there's more than five. I'm expanding my sixth,
    which has been explosive as dynamite.

Plus, the study of astrology, tarot,
    and other metaphysical disciplines
Has stretched my awareness of self and others,
    revealing what's hiding within our origins.

It's taught me to be less hateful and filling up
    with guilt toward my sugar imbalances.
For further healing, I'm exploring the deeper,
    hidden meanings of my life's circumstances.

As I am learning to heighten all of my senses,
    due to the sight sense being too weak,
I've kept most my students perplexed, especially
    those unruly ones who were not so meek.

In using my third eye, I'd catch a student
    misbehaving in the back of my classroom.
The student would ask me in awe, "I thought
    you couldn't see?" as I began to lower the boom.

I would respond, "You would be surprised what I can
    and can't see,"Beaming, being quite satisfied
As he uncomfortably begins to squirm in his seat,
    feeling bewildered and stupefied.

Normally, I'm confident, but I was nervous
    to have my teaching evaluated
By my narrow-minded boss due to my vision,
    where I was horribly discriminated.

I instructed, "Grab your books." One student
    refusing to move, saying, "I don't have my book."
Unable to see it, I requested with assuredness,
    "It's under your desk, take a look."

I, sometimes, have an overabundance of confidence,
    relying on my in-tune gut.
This keeps my students guessing after observing me daily
    and hearing some school scuttlebutt.

My watchful boss and students were either baffled
    or assumed I could easily see it.
My intuition was helpful, preventing others
    from labeling me as being unfit.

It's puzzling to others as well as to me,
    how I can't see well, including small print.
Then occasionally, I am somehow capable of spotting
    some insignificant lint.

I'm a concrete sequential, rely on good memory,
    and use my personal sonar.
Besides being organized and storing items properly,
    this has all guided me so far.

With things in order, I just want to reach out
    and grab, relying on my impaired eyes less.
I'll alphabetize, spring clean, use color tape,
    and label, keeping all in an orderly mess.

Low vision has been teaching me to use my six senses.
    This also includes my third eye.
Many folks are still unaware or do not wish to accept,
    and sadly, they choose to deny.

It's subtle, but when I get a hunch or a light feeling,
    my blood sugar levels are low.
I don't always listen since my logical mind
    is much bolder and will often tell me, "No."

The logical mind sticks around.
    It is not as accurate as one's intuitive voice.
It gives more time to be analytical or critical,
    causing one to make a poor choice.

My inner voice comes in flashes,
    is accurate, and often speaks in another tone.
I'm learning to distinguish between the two,
    not realizing this until I was fully grown.

Here is an example of mixing and confusing
    my intuition with my logic.
Reminding me if I am uncertain or lack trust,
    it may draw me to events that could be tragic.

Like eating baked chicken, green salad with lemon juice,
    brown rice, and cabbage for dinnertime.
Then two and a half hours later, my glucose is 92.
    It's good, but too close to bedtime.

Within sixty minutes, I'd then hear this little voice
    swirling around in my sleepy head
To please check your blood sugar level, it's spiraling down,
    before turning the lights off for bed.

One Starburst will raise my sugars.
    This drop wasn't surprising, but can be expected.
I awoke with 196, so need to stay attentive.
    My regulating can improve, but not be perfected.

I'll eat well and keep in shape,
    since keeping on top of my diabetes can be wearing.
This just gives more importance to exercising,
    so I can feel good to want to keep caring.

Plus, I can't forget the times where both my ears
    must stay flapping, deemphasizing logic.
Relying more on those mysterious voices,
    carrying what seems like a touch of magic.

Once, I left my insulin at home.
    My husband was preparing to travel out of state.
My inner voice urged me to call him,
    However, my logical mind said I was much too late.

He first drove a friend to Seattle. My inner voice whispered,
    call the friend, leave a message.
With the universe's help, my supplies were soon delivered,
    free via a psychic expressage.

I was thankful he heard my cry for help in time
	as he was traveling a great distance.
He was restless and wanted to get going
	right after he first came to his friend's assistance.

Feeling some heat, the cooks assured me
	both ovens were off as I glanced at unclear dials.
The next day, I asked chef's sister and husband
	to double-check. One was on, my feeling sense smiles.

In this particular case, I didn't need to use
	my insightful eyes, impaired or not.
Why the other two sighted chefs didn't feel the warmth
	or see the dials on was strange I thought.

Using my feeling and hearing, I was standing
	near our unattended gas stove burner.
The unknown dancing flame could be harmful.
	I need to keep alert, being an aware learner.

When I am preparing fresh fruit like washing
	and slicing grapes and strawberries for my meals.
I can't tell by looking at it if it's rotten,
	but my fingers clue me in to how it feels.

When I'm out walking, my feet are more sensitive
	to the ground's varying sloping surface.
Then, there are times my body's unexpectedly jolted,
	which could lead to being treacherous.

Once my husband and I were lost,
	looking for an escalator in a department store.
He relies heavily on sight, but says,
	"Oh no, my 20/20 isn't working any more."

Hearing the humming of the escalator, I pointed,
    "This way." He points, "No, it's this way."
Since my husband sees well, I rely more on him,
    listening closely to what he has to say.

I was unaware at first I had used my ears
    to help guide us in the right direction.
If one can't see, it's not bizarre to automatically use
    other means for detection.

While shopping, I ask, "How much is this?" Larry shrugs,
    "Don't know." I ask, "What does the sign say?"
He replies, after looking everywhere, "Why are you so smart?"
    as the price is clearly displayed.

Thus, it's not all intuition,
    but a common selling practice which is ordinary.
A sign centered among items for sale,
    an everyday selling routine that's customary.

Dreams are fantasies, fears, and premonitions,
    drawing on supernatural dimension.
Dreams are our subconscious, giving us
    important messages that require our attention.

I dreamt once of having a low blood sugar,
    struggling, then I was abruptly awake.
I laid there for a second, wondering its meaning,
    then got up for my routine bathroom break.

I was unable to relieve myself easily,
    all pointing toward a low sugar cue.
Yes, my sugar level was forty-one, telling me
    to grab juice and a soft candy fruit chew.

What does my future foresee
*   as I'm guided on my fated journey?*

My journey is bittersweet.
    I am finally realizing my potential is limitless.
I just needed to change my shortsighted attitude
    in needing a little more willingness.

My mind is expanding beyond horizons
    that I never knew existed.
Imagine how far I'd be if I had a clue,
    or I hadn't previously resisted.

Our perception of reality is far greater
    than what we previously believed.
To enhance sight, I must identify my gifts,
    trusting spiritual guidance I receive.

Spirituality begins deeply inside us,
    a personal inward perception.
I need to keep honest, especially with myself,
    avoiding any sort of deception.

As I turn my medical challenges into gifts,
    I'm realizing I'm not cursed, but blessed.
Allowing myself to be seen in a new, bright light,
    growing and evolving in consciousness.

Through what I have learned and experienced,
    I wish to share, hoping it helps society.
As my destined path unfolds, I'll find my hidden self
    through studies of spirituality.

We are surrounded by life's lessons
through the people we meet and our experiences.
I believe there is a Divine Order to our life.
There's no such thing as coincidences.

Chapter VII

After considering all things, it is a short, 24-inch "leash,"
   my new lease on life.
My insulin pump does help me daily to experience
   a lot less diabetic strife.

My body and I were very tired of taking five shots,
   sometimes six to manage a day.
Both of us feeling blessedly lucky and grateful
   that the insulin pump has come our way.

The impact or value was clearly shown through my A1Cs
   as they've improved a great deal.
Furthermore, I now can be less rigid, having more freedom
   when I choose to eat a meal.

If my brittle blood sugar levels are too high
   or too low, and yes, they certainly are.
It is much easier to keep my sugar levels in balance.
   At least, it has been so far.

One advantage is I no longer need to give myself
   a whole unit, two, three, or more.
Now, I can fine-tune the insulin amounts,
   like bolusing point-9, 1-point--2, or point-4.

After considering all things, it is a short, 24-inch "leash,"
    my new lease on life.
My insulin pump does help me daily to experience
    a lot less diabetic strife.

These researchers deserve much praise
    for inventing this pump, truly gifted geniuses.
The pump's a battery-operated microprocessor,
    close to a healthy pancreas.

It automatically gives me
    an hourly, predetermined dose of insulin.
Each three minutes I'll get a percentage of that.
    It sure beats using a syringe discipline.

Before I eat, mainly carbohydrates,
    or if my glucose is elevated too high,
I will bolus myself additional insulin.
    It sure beats a syringe shot in my thigh.

However, if my glucose level is a scary high,
    teetering on the extreme side,
I will gladly give myself a syringe shot,
    hoping my sweetened blood will begin to subside.

One of my pump's features I find most beneficial
    is the temporary basal rate.
Insulin can be raised or lowered in 10% increments.
    It's simple to calculate.

It is especially effective for exercising, illness,
    or when having surgery.
Of course, I still need to keep a close eye on my blood
    so it does not become too sugary.

Can pumpers play the peek-a-boo game?
Our pumps aren't all worn exactly the same.

On the more challenging or more irritable side,
    is having the pump always nearby.
Yet, the pros definitely do outweigh the few cons,
    which helps to keep me feeling satisfied.

Obviously, for the insulin pump to work well,
    it needs to be connected to me.
Thus, it gives me an occasional restrictive feeling
    of not being absolutely free.

There are alternative ways with or without accessories
    to wear the insulin pump.
However, no matter where the pump is connected,
    it appears or is felt like a small lump.

The pump can even be hidden from view
    by strapping it to one's thigh, high above the knee.
It'd help if one's wearing a revealing cocktail dress,
    a perfect spot, since nobody can see.

Some like to stash their pump in their pocket.
    Yet, a lot also depends on one's body size.
It'd be accessible, but too uncomfortable for me.
    This position I would despise.

I've tried stuffing it in my sports bra,
    like when wearing a bulky, loosely-fitted sweater.
Perhaps, if I were more endowed and wouldn't bend over,
    this position would work much better.

Throughout my everyday activities,
    what I have personally found that works best
Is keeping the pump in a bra pouch under my arm
    that is hooked to my bra next to my chest.

Then the pump is out of sight and out of the way,
    and my pump doesn't feel like such a pest.
So, for the most part, no matter what I wear,
    it really doesn't interfere with how I'm dressed.

At night, however, it is not as easy
    if not clipped to me, which for me is handy.
It can easily be lost, until my hubby turns over
    and shrieks, "Ouch! What is hurting me?"

Or when I roll out of bed, my husband
    will jokingly remind me, "Don't forget your tail!"
I will frustratingly find it, grab it, and cry out
    in a loud, booming voice, "Oh, what the hell!"

Painfully, there are times the site is pulled out,
    which of course doesn't feel so well.
I just need to keep reminding myself my life could be worse.
    There is no good reason to yell.

Does the pump hinder my sexual appetite?
    Does it keep me under-sexed and uptight?

When I was introduced to the pump,
    sex was actually one of my first silent thoughts.
Visualizing the inconveniences, weighing the idea
    of those less agonizing shots.

There is still sex after insulin pump
    for those who have a lustful and curious mind.
The pump can stay clipped to you or not, hoping
    you don't get wound awkwardly into a bind.

I must keep adapting my lifestyle,
    keeping creative, flexible, and open minded.
My priorities in life are ever changing.
    Life is good. I don't need to be reminded.

Which infusion set is right for me?
    Is there such a thing as being pain free?

Through the process of elimination,
    I use the infusion set, the Rapid-D-6.
I have tried using for months the Ultra Flex
    and the Tender, the other two possible picks.

Every six days I must change part of my infusion set.
    I call it my "leash" or hose.
They're 24, 31, or 43 inches long,
    the longest reaching close to my toes.

I change the needle of my infusion set
    every two days, not spontaneously.
It needs time to heal, where the stainless steel needle
    has been inserted subcutaneously.

This prevents scar tissue from building up
    so insulin can be absorbed and it won't sit.
The muscle near the belly button affects the absorption, too,
    so one must stay clear of it.

We're not the same, but I'll stay two inches away,
    keep rotating, or problems may occur.
Therefore, I'll use my tender stomach, hips, legs,
    and my upper arms, rotating my site for sure.

The infusion set that is less desirable,
    or least preferred, is the Rapid-D.
Through the trials of the three infusion sets,
    the Rapid-D has been working the best for me.

Some dislike its short "tail," stainless steel needle,
    and how its parts are changed, making it more complex.
The most widely used one or sought after infusion set
    for most pumpers is the Ultra Flex.

The Teflon cannula is most used
    with its short introducer needle to help insert.
Like with most needles, it pierces the skin painlessly
    and quickly. It often does not hurt.

Plus, I liked rotating three days apart,
    and the 90 degree angle, pushing straight in.
Yet, my tough skin kept bending the needle or cannula
    and the tape irritated my skin.

It was comfortable and easy to connect at the site,
    hearing an audible click.
I was disappointed this infusion set didn't work.
    It would have been my favorite pick.

Next, I tried using the Tender set,
    which also has a Teflon cannula for comfort.
It easily slides into a base with an audible click,
    attaching it takes little effort.

A three day rotation, but the insertion
    was in a 30-45-degree angle.
It's tough to do alone. My mate wanted
    to grab the tubing, wrap it around me, and strangle.

It would take many stabs to get it right;
    besides needles bending; I was in misery.
Having no choice again, this is how I was led
    to my least favorite, the Rapid-D.

I wasn't looking forward to a stainless steel needle,
    fearing how comfortable it'd be.
I had to try before my imagination went wild,
    but there was one advantage for me.

Inserting a needle at right angles
    is much easier to do when I must self-stick.
Besides, with the "tail," I can reach spots on my backside.
    It's now becoming a much better pick.

I'm adjusting to the stainless steel needle
    and the "tail" left hanging loosely from my site.
So far, it's comfortable and simple,
    the end of my disheartening infusion set plight.

Either it's me, or when my Dr. Hubby helps,
    one can hear from a distance, a few loud yelps.

When my non-diabetic husband lends a hand,
    he's stabbed mistakenly on occasion.
He has had his share in dealing with a few
    too many unwanted pokes and some abrasions.

There was one night when he was assisting me,
    filling my syringe shot while lying in bed.
Somehow, in our exchange, it slipped from my hands,
    sticking into his bare chest, just missing his head.

It looked like a perfect human Bull's Eye;
    my husband let out a fierce, startled, painful yelp.
We need to be more careful and be alert the next time
    or he may no longer choose to help.

Now and then, when he helps me change my needle
    for a new sterile one in my autolet,
I will suddenly hear a wailing shriek,
    reacting as if he's been stabbed by a bayonet.

My loving mate can be over dramatic for a few sharp pokes,
    barely piercing his skin.
It is difficult for me to give much sympathy,
    not I, the pin cushion, Cheryl Lynn.

For showering, I'll remove my pump, and once
    when I was ready to be reconnected.
I panicked on our boat, silently thinking,
    oh no, my husband will again be dissected.

My needle and the "little tail" of my Rapid-D-6
    was missing, causing an alarm,
Leaving only a partial part of the round tape
    still attached to the upper part of my arm.

Frantically searching for the missing needle,
    not in my arm, the boat's head, or our bed,
I shook vigorously and repeatedly our pillows, sheets,
    blankets, and our queen-size bedspread.

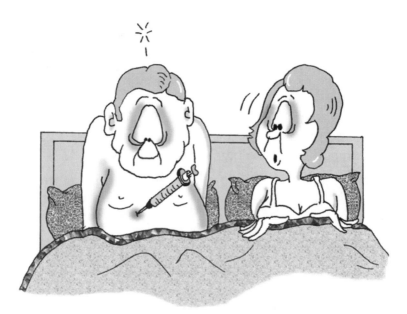

Having no such luck, I gave my Captain
  a warning of a possible painful surprise.
He needed to be attentive and keep a sharp watch out
  for another sharp needle demise.

It had snagged on our electrical panel door
  in our shower without me giving a shout.
Our shower's narrow and I'm surprised it wasn't felt
  as I was twirling and twisting about.

I was shocked. It causes pain if hooked on a doorknob,
  pulling down my pants, or if caught on anything.
My "leash" doesn't always stay well hidden.
  It is like I'm tethered to an annoying long string.

Today, it may look suspicious,
  living post-9/11, having it partly hang out.
I don't dare joke, "Beware, I'm connected to a bomb!"
  Someone may panic and began to shout.

But on innumerable occasions, I'll have a loop
  slip out from underneath my clothes.
I use the shortest "leash," but this is how it's often snagged,
  which can cause me to fall on my nose.

This worries me to lose even one, fearing
  my medical pump supplies will run too low.
And my insurance requires me to replace lost supplies
  at my own expense, what a blow.

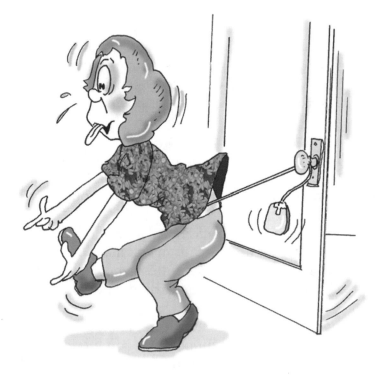

I can get angry and be steaming hot
  if I don't know my pump's working or not.

Every now and then, when my brittle sugar levels
    are unstable, far out of whack,
I will drink lots of water. But I can't allow myself to eat,
    not even a little snack.

The longest food fast lasted a miserable two whole days,
    too long of a time to wait.
My body must have really paid. I know this certainly is
    an improper way to lose weight.

Normally, it does not take me as long
    to get my blood sugars back to the proper range.
Moreover, it is often my insulin pump
    when my blood sugar levels are acting strange.

If my pump isn't working properly, it may beep,
    being explained by its many codes.
I can use my back-up pump or resort to
    syringe shots for such unbearable episodes.

I need to troubleshoot by changing my infusion set
    with a brand new Rapid-D-6.
Perhaps the site's infected, the tubing's pinched,
    or scar tissue, but this usually does the trick.

Thus, it is trial and error as the answers
    are not always obvious or that clear.
I can only hope that such irregularities
    are a rarity to deal with each year.

Do any medical insurance programs
    cover these unscheduled required changes?
Well, not according to my own inquiries,
    one's not allotted these type of exchanges.

If insurance companies had rising high blood sugars,
    how would they like to handle this?
I'm just curious, can't give any extra supplies
    for such incidents that could go amiss.

I must admit the company, not my insurance,
    has sent me a few extra supplies.
There are limits and this makes me insecure.
    I'd rather buy low-vision tools for my impaired eyes.

Besides a back-up pump, it is reassuring
    there's a 1-800 number to call.
It's available 24 hours for any pump questions,
    gladly, it includes nightfall.

Technicians are standing by who have been
    patient, knowledgeable, and ready to assist.
They've helped me in solving my panic situations,
    so my pump problems no longer persist.

The warning beeping sounds continuously beep
    until I figure out what's going on.
I usually first will think it is a commercial truck
    backing up, taking much, much too long.

Once on our boat, the beeping sounds
    became irritating, trying to clue me in.
The beeps are endless until the problem is corrected,
    leaving me in a searching whirlwind.

I kept hearing this annoying constant beeping sound
  wherever I went.
Looked in the engine room, the gauges
  even slowed down, much time was being spent.

After a few hours, I found out
  it's not the boat, but me!
It was my insulin pump, trying to tell me
  a low battery![1]

Some insulin pumps have the option to vibrate
  if there's a problem until it's resolved.
Whether it vibrates or beeps, it can't be ignored.
  Action must be taken; one must get involved.

Just throw me an old gunnysack.
  I'll stash my supplies into one raggedy pack.

No matter where we go, it's not easy to pack light,
  traveling to our special places.
My husband wants to pack only one bag,
  but we end up taking at least three full suitcases.

One suitcase is filled with diabetic supplies,
  including extras for emergencies.
Whether it is a short or long trip, one can see,
  packing for me causes great difficulties.

Here's a sample list: blood sugar meter,
  glucose strips, autolet, lancets, this is not all.
Glucose Control Solutions, alcohol wipes, cotton balls,
  and batteries, ready to install.

---

1. excerpt from *Alaska Bound On The Cheryl Lynn, A Mariner's Rhyming Log* by Cheryl Lynn

A diary for recording results, a pen,
    all tucked in my meter case, yes, there's more.
Insulin, syringes, my pump, back-up pump,
    and Glucagon, if out in the tules, at least four

Pump batteries, piston rod, cartridges filling needles,
    pump adapter, yes, the list goes on.
Infusion sets, antiseptic wipes, protective cap,
    manual. Tired yet, ready to yawn?

Having diabetes can be a disturbing fact.
    My pump helps to keep my mind and body intact.

Overall, my pump has had a positive effect,
    as balance is my ultimate aim.
The insulin pump isn't the answer for everyone.
    Our needs, of course, aren't always the same.

There are so many more good points that,
    without a doubt, definitely do outweigh the bad.
I must always keep looking through positive impaired eyes,
    not allowing myself to feel sad.

The challenging side of dealing with diabetes
    isn't always easy to accept.
For us to reach personal happiness,
    we must be capable of improving our mindset.

If I harbor destructive impulses or
    negative thoughts toward me or society,
How could I possibly heal myself
    if I am burdened with such deep, heavy anxiety?

With gathering together my husband, pump, vigilance,
    and being able to self-stick,
I am healthier, happy, and balanced
    despite having a disease that's brittle and chronic.

Most importantly, I've found it is vital
    in taking numerous blood glucose self-tests.
This self-monitoring is essential to my well-being,
    so I can keep feeling my best.

There's a tremendous, long list of worse medical challenges
    I could be suffering from.
By being consciously aware of this disturbing fact,
    it does keep me from feeling so glum.

If I look at the big picture, having diabetes
    isn't so dreadful, one can cope.
It is a manageable struggle, and there's a chance for a cure.
    Therefore, there's at least some hope.

Most people don't get away in dealing with medical issues,
    keeping healthy and sound.
Some are afflicted more than their fair share,
    early or later in life, just take a look around.

Chapter VIII

I am willing and try to keep an open mind
  to whatever research might someday find.
It may work to one's advantage to be a guinea pig.
  I'm waiting for the next brilliant mind.

I am willing and try to keep an open mind
  to whatever research might someday find.
It may work to one's advantage to be a guinea pig.
  I'm waiting for the next brilliant mind.

Medical researchers use countless trial and error,
  delaying us before we buy.
Trials can go on after a purchase.
  My Gluco-Watch G2 Biographer went awry.

Its incessant alarm would sound if my blood sugar levels
  were too high or spooky low.
Its idea was fabulous and would have given comfort
  whether relaxed or on the go.

The Gluco-Watch used batteries and was worn
  on my wrist like wearing a simple watchband.
It measured one's glucose levels through the skin,
  but unfortunately, it did not work as planned.

Failures are bound to happen, which makes me hope
    that insurance companies' concerns are met.
We rely on their continual support.
    We hope there are no future feelings of regret.

Researchers have not given up on this idea.
    It is being improved and fine-tuned.
There's a new product used with or without one's pump.
    More diabetics will be using one soon.

It's called a Continuous Glucose Monitor
    or CGM, an effective device.
It measure's one's glucose every five minutes,
    the long-term health benefits outweighs the price.

It can detect patterns and trends in one's glucose levels
    to help tighten up one's control.
An alarm alerts one if the glucose drops
    or rises outside the targeted glucose goal.

I was given the chance to try it for a week.
    It is a step in the right direction.
My skin area for sites has limited real estate.
    This calls for another injection.

My insulin pump does not work with it,
    so my pump and monitor were worn on each hip.
I felt like Wyatt Earp with his gunslinger holster,
    ready to fire, letting bullets rip.

Sensors are changed three days apart.
    They are injected into one's body's fatty tissue.
Mine bled when it was first inserted and had to be replaced.
    This could be a costly issue.

Some insurance still needs to be convinced.
　A few have been approved and supplies authorized.
Insurances must see greater savings with blood testing
　and how the cost would be minimized..

My second sensor was pulled out in two days.
　My husband thinks they are for the inactive.
Yet, the third one worked without me slowing down.
　I remained my busy self and I kept active.

It showed my blood sugar levels were running
　too high between two to six in the a.m..
Thus, my doctor raised my basal rates slightly.
　Gaining tighter control makes this product a gem.

This trial was an exhausting week for not only me,
　but also for my good husband.
Benefits could be far reaching for us
　and our caretakers, there is help for everyone.

At this time, diabetics have just a few
　Continuous Glucose Monitors to choose.
Since I'm brittle, a day shouldn't pass without wearing a CGM;
　I have nothing to lose.

Before the insulin pump, when pen needles were introduced,
　I was more than eager to try.
I tried two different ones, both pen needles worked well,
　grateful my insurance did not deny.

Filling a syringe with failing eyesight was hard,
　trusting, I was accurate and precise.
Yet, I could click off units and insert an insulin cartridge
　into a pen-like device.

They've invented a device to slip onto the syringe,
  magnifying so one can read.
Its strength wasn't enough for me, a stronger hand-held,
  lighted magnifier is what I need.

How would our lives be
without technology?

Without the significant, ever increasing
  advancements of technology,
I, personally, can't even begin to imagine
  how my diabetic life would be.

Over the last years, research for diabetes
  and medicine has certainly advanced.
It gives us hope in how we'll manage, knowing
  our condition will improve and soon be enhanced.

Progress is moving swiftly, look how times have changed,
  like with the meaning of the word mouse.
As a kid, I would first think of Mickey Mouse or
  a rodent in the barn or in our house.

In today's updated society, think,
  what would first come to mind with our progeny?
It is the computer mouse, living in a computerized world
  with all of its technology.

The benefits of technology have helped my diabetes.
  It has greatly improved.
With newer insulin, glucose monitors, pumps,
  plus, waiting for more products to be approved.

To self-test, I'm grateful for the glucose monitors,
    instead of using urine test strips.
It is easier to dine out, be active, and travel,
    packing less bulky supplies for trips.

The availability of sugar free foods
    and awareness of how food affects you;
The different implements one can use to inject a shot
    just keeps getting better. Yahoo!

Plus, low vision tools are being developed as I write;
    makes me eager for a new "toy".
We low visual aid users count on progress
    so we can better enjoy.

Research is on the cutting edge of great ideas,
    making exciting, new improvements.
What a great hi-tech world we live in,
    with ongoing promising beneficial developments.

Eating healthy can be a chore.
    It doesn't have to be a bore.

In the beginning days in learning what I could eat,
    it was hard finding sugar free food.
It was extremely difficult for me to keep smiling
    or to stay in a bright, cheerful mood.

As I sat down for nourishment at mealtimes,
    scowling over my healthier tasteless meal,
Not having any of my old time favorites,
    it didn't give me much of the same appeal.

Sadly, both grapes and watermelon were then,
    no longer allowed on my grocery list.
Being such a fruit lover, those were two fruits
    with too high sugar content I knew I'd miss.

To eat healthy took too much effort and work,
    weighing, measuring, and buying my own scale,
Figuring out the calories and quantities,
    and still not being allowed just one cocktail.

I was shocked how small a 150 gram apple looked
    as well as other foodstuff.
It wasn't fun being the cook in my kitchen,
    mastering my diabetic diet was tough.

Through this, I have become accustomed to counting
    all the carbohydrates, fats, and proteins.
It just took me awhile to readjust. I now stay on the lookout
    for new eating routines.

At our family functions, many were considerate
    and thoughtful of my special diet.
Plus, we had experimental salt and wheat-free meals
    for those in need spread across our dinette.

My disenchanted brother in a half-serious
    and half-teasing way would always quiz,
"Where's the human food?" not wanting to be fooled
    by these creative meals, just wanting his.

Research has created many artificial sweeteners.
    Today there is a whole bunch.
Depending how the sweeteners are used, some work
    and some don't, of course, there isn't the same punch.

With one of the first artificial sugars,
    my mom baked some brownies, hoping I'd be pleased.
My friend joined us, as we were all curious,
    but our taste buds were displeased.

First, the anticipating taste test caused much laughter,
    reducing to disappointing tears.
It was disgusting, especially after eating
    regular sugar for so many years.

Nowadays, my husband can make a yummy apple pie
    that can add a smile to one's face.
He uses Equal and many of our friends do not know
    or can tell and still enjoy the taste.

Throughout the years, I've tried many sweeteners
    including using apple juice and honey.
Of course, special foods for varying diets
    and some with less ingredients cost more money.

Homemade applesauce with only apples and water,
    no additives is what I prefer.
I, too, like buying, without question, canned fruit,
    chicken, or tuna fish packed in water for sure.

I eat sugarless cereal with nonfat milk;
    my taste buds have learned to be adaptive.
On my own, I make these healthier choices,
    not allowing my diet to hold me captive.

Some sugar-free candies have a much higher fat content,
    a fact to consider and weigh.
I'll take note of the sugar substitution;
    some I'll disagree with, while others are okay.

Sugar alcohols like sorbitol, mannitol,
    any ending in ol, must not eat tons.
These sugar substitutes can cause gastric disturbances,
    in giving one possibly the runs.

I'm no angel and eat foods not on my healthy grocery list,
    I have my cheating ways.
Thanks to research, it's easier now to make better food choices
    than in the earlier days.

Researchers have found creative substitutions
    for many foods, like various cheeses,
Lactose, cholesterol, and salt-free,
    or varying fat content designed for most diseases.

A few may not taste the best, but can be eaten
    if one's cheesy taste buds need to be pleased.
The cooks may partially satisfy cheese lovers
    by concocting ingenious recipes.

When my husband and I fix ourselves something
    hot to drink on a cold bitter, wintry day,
We will frequently choose sugar-free hot chocolate,
    which thanks to research, has come a long way.

Please do not think that I am complaining,
    but my hot chocolate drink does look rather thin.
Lucky for me, I should be delighted and elated,
    it is sugar-free for Cheryl Lynn.

Even years ago in trying to manage
    and keep my diabetes under control,
My doctor advised me to eat sugar.
    I was tickled, ready to dance around the Maypole.

This was during the time when sugar was forbidden,
    it was absolutely not allowed.
Curiosity led me to check an hour or two afterward,
    sugars weren't bad, Oh, Wow!

I have learned my sugars increase
    if I eat potatoes, pizza, and such carbohydrates.
Not as much when eating candy and desserts
    is what my sugar level for me indicates.

It's now easier to balance with my pump
    when I choose to sparingly eat something sweet.
On the other hand, fat calories remain,
    adding to my whole body from head to my feet.

Still, today, it's rough managing my insulin intake,
    particularly at parties.
The timing, watching quantities, and being surrounded by
    tempting snacks and many goodies.

Thanks again, through research, eating sugar
    is more acceptable for us than it once was.
Moderation, a watchful eye, and self-testing
    are needed to see just what the sugar does.

There are daily updated nutritional facts
    for all sorts of medical disorders.
Earlier on, diet pop was threatened.
    Many scrambled in a panic and became hoarders.

There's an ongoing debate on what's good for you or not,
    moderation is always the key.
Individuals must make up their own mind,
    listening to their bodies' cries most carefully.

Staying healthy is the key.
Is alternative medicine for me?

I feel, try traditional and nontraditional avenues
    and research on one's own.
We never know what problems we may help or cure
    in healing ourselves from the strange and unknown.

Thus, I sought out a Naturopathic,
    following his specialized diet to a tee.
I ended up in a coma three times in one week.
    This obviously wasn't helping me.

The same medics, recognizing my address,
    came each time to my rescue and brought me to.
I even slept at my sister's for more help.
    The medics smiled, instantly knowing what to do.

An ingredient had to be eliminated,
    pressuring me to bake my own bread.
Plus, too much diet change can affect one's sugars.
    This time we were just unknowingly misled.

We all respond differently to insulin
    and the quantity of what we must take.
Another diabetic might take twice as much insulin
    as I for the same food intake.

It can be helpful to network with friends
    for ideas to make recovery speedy.
In healing infections on my feet or hands,
    I use the Spacey Lacy, a home remedy.

My girlfriend's father used it on his feet
    before they were about to be amputated.
It saved his feet from surgery.
    The infection miraculously was eliminated.

After much money and numerous trips to a special clinic,
    his feet were not healing.
He was discouraged and willing to try anything
    to save his feet so they could keep feeling.

He tried an unorthodox cure
    by soaking his feet in Epsom salt water for a bit.
Then placing aloe vera and sugar on his feet
    and wrapping bandages upon it.

Twice a day her father would change his bandages,
    grinning as the infection slowly healed.
As unbelievable as it might sound, his feet were saved
    and how he did it, he kept concealed.

Amazing, this ancient cure costs near a buck fifty
    and is found in his kitchen canisters.
Such feet saving rewards, he'll be keeping an eye
    on any cuts, burns, open sores, or blisters.

In self-doctoring with this healing concoction,
    and in treating for an infected wound,
I'd soak, sit with sugar and aloe vera for at least 20 minutes.
    It, too, heals soon.

The aloe vera plant is known for its healing qualities,
    one should be in each home.
I'll cut some pieces from our plant before my husband and I
    take off for a few days to roam.

The sugar is like using raw or pasteurized honey
    according to some other friends.
They say it draws the toxins out, kills the bacteria,
    as it hastens the healing and mends.

As a result, networking did pay off.
    Sugar and honey may work as healing agents.
If this unscientific method had not worked out,
    one would be missing only a few cents.

Research costs,
    however, without it, we'd be lost.

A researcher told me once it cost less than a penny
    to produce each blood sugar strip.
Does that make sense with such exorbitant prices
    at what diabetics must pay? What a rip!

Are these outrageous prices greed,
    or is it what our researchers need in their search?
The degree of profit may be too high,
    However, it's used for development and research.

I want a balance between the lowest paid employees
    and the CEO's own profit.
Leaving enough revenue to discover products,
    since we need and do appreciate it.

In most businesses, big or small,
    we need individuals with profit-seeking concerns.
As long as this isn't their main focal point
    and can serve us with honest financial returns.

There is a fine line or a wide gray area
    between the net gain and those into greed.
Plus, there are thousands of workers finding employment,
    which is what our economy does need.

Thus, it gets costly if one must deal with an illness
    and in getting the proper treatments.
A future medical issue we hope our country can solve
    as we wait for new improvements.

However, if we're going to be sick,
    nowadays is a better time than in our past.
With the latest technology, people are much healthier
    and for many more years can last.

Some have stated, if it weren't for my personality
    and technology, I'd be dead.
It's, perhaps, true, encouraging me to live a full life,
    dreaming of new products up ahead.

Chapter IX

If some of our unsound, poorer choices are
hanging us up, we need to set ourselves free.
Withdraw, reflect, to ask what needs to be cleared
away, so there's new growth and fresh energy.

There are an alarming, growing number
of individuals who are diabetic.
Diabetes Millitus is rapidly increasing.
It's becoming an epidemic.

Many people share our same experiences.
We are not alone as we think we are.
It is healing to give voice to our feelings with others,
so we're not leaving ourselves a scar.

My mind's on overload, too much mental processing.
Its active gears are always turning.
Can a diabetic ever flick the switch off for peace
and do some relaxing sojourning?

It's such a juggling act, with emotional
and physical demands, in how we eat,
Making sure we keep our minds clear of toxic thoughts,
exercise, and pay attention to our feet.

We must wear socks, shouldn't go barefoot,
    watch out for any cuts or wounds. Can I take this pill?
If I close my eyes, will I wake up on my own,
    concerns during surgery, or if I'm ill.

How are both of my kidneys, my heart?
    Will my eyes be impaired due to retinopathy?
One may worry about slow healing, amputation,
    nerve damage leading to neuropathy.

If I eat this, do this activity, and watch the time,
    will my blood sugars be okay?
How will I carry my snacks, glucose meter,
    and how often must I check my sugars today?

If desired, paths will start opening up
    to reach out to those sharing the same health issues,
Emailing, web surfing, chat rooms, support groups,
    and reading bulletins are a few avenues.

Born with spunk, boldness, and stick-to-it-iveness,
    traits that have been an asset throughout my life,
Whether things are going well for me, a friendly competition,
    or health, or domestic strife.

My doctors and husband recognize
    this bulldog tenacity in everything I do.
How it's enhanced my diabetes management,
    other health issues, or my daily life too.

It does help to have such sheer determination
    and be focused in wanting to excel.
Many of my friends who understand me know
    I will rarely give up and say, "Oh what the hell!"

Perhaps it wasn't good, struggling so long
    with the unknown symptoms as I persevered.
Besides, the medical practitioners didn't help,
    leaving me always feeling miserable and weird.

We must take charge, keep getting involved,
    not relying solely on our caretakers,
Despite our shyness, fears, laziness, or busy lifestyles
    as professionals or homemakers.

Nowadays, it's helping to expand my intuition
    and how sensitive I've become.
In addition, having a doting, sharp-eyed husband,
    who keeps me close under his caring thumb.

Even though my husband has tendencies
    to getting grouchy, impatient, and a bit tense,
He just worries too much in taking care of me,
    ready for a diabetic incidence.

My insulin pump and husband have enhanced
    my daily control of my diabetes.
Plus, taking numerous blood sugar self-tests,
    are all helping me in mastering this disease.

Most importantly, my attitude and outlook on life
    have grown and changed for the better.
As well as my commitment to not feel sorry for myself,
    to give up, or be a quitter.

I'm overcoming anger, hatred, and deciding
    to meet my diabetes halfway.
I'm striving for fulfillment, not perfection,
    showing a healthier emotional display.

Yes, for some universal reason,
    I still do get the unwanted sugar highs and lows.
Yet, luckily for me, not as many erratic sugar levels,
    as I did once ago.

I am aware that some diabetic complications
    could definitely still occur.
I'll keep my spirits high and my fingers crossed,
    for I've already dealt with my fair share for sure.

No longer do I question why my sugars
    don't match some diabetics as they tell me.
I've finally quit asking, "Why can't that be me?"
    realizing acceptance is a crucial key.

Some are opinionated and freely give
    their medical or nonmedical advice.
One must understand all diabetics can be different,
    it's not a disease that's concise.

Even though the basic concepts, medical supplies,
    and the outcomes can all be the same,
I must keep reminding myself not to allow others
    to make me feel like I am to blame.

Not so much today, but the medical field
    did squeeze us all into the same health chapter.
Now beginning to realize what works for one
    doesn't work for all, and this they need to factor.

Our diets need to be tailored to our individual lifestyles
    and who we uniquely are.
Blood sugar results can differ even if two diabetics
    eat the same chocolate bar.

However, I've always said this world would be boring
　　if we all drove blue Volkswagens.
I must remember, we're all uniquely different.
　　We do not follow the same regimen.

Why can't we have enough faith and complete trust,
　　to take charge of our health to do what we must?
What is it that keeps blocking us? Are we being fair
　　to our bodies? Are we being unjust?

In keeping on the road to good health,
　　it'd help to make regular visits to one's doctor.
If unable to drive, find a true friend, use Access,
　　or hail a taxi, if not a walker.

Before my scheduled visits, I'll scribble out a list
　　in German of my questions to ask.
This helps me from forgetting any details,
　　besides keeping us both focused, staying on task.

Why do we procrastinate, dragging both our feet
　　to make an appointment with our doctors?
And for a few stubborn folks,
　　why does it take fear to be one of the motivating factors?

I've even met diabetics who have noticed vision loss,
　　refusing to see someone.
They are avoiding a painless eye exam,
　　perhaps, fearing problems have already begun.

In the real world, our doctors or we can't always be successful.
　　We must accept this fact.
It doesn't mean one should stop trying.
　　One needs to do what one can to keep one's body intact.

Why aren't we scared to eat at fast food drive-ins,
    cross the street, rise out of bed, and face the day,
Or get into a car mishap or boating collision,
    and need to radio MAYDAY?

Life for me takes self-discipline, focus,
    and effort, being a brittle diabetic.
However, I still find ways to enjoy life to the fullest,
    making me more energetic.

There are times when I'm irritated,
    wanting to ignore it all, finding a hole to hide.
Yet, each diabetic day is teaching me it won't pay.
    There's not a whole lot of room to slide.

It's important to stay committed to our health issues,
    to be triumphant for each day.
I'll summon inner strength, using sheer determination
    to conquer obstacles in my way.

During my life, I am trying to overcome the odds
    and confront my competition.
I need to keep the strength and tenacity
    to stand up to such powerful opposition.

If you cannot do it on your own,
    seek out your very own encouraging cheerleader.
One needs to reach out, make a call, and ask,
    not everyone at times can be a psychic reader.

The bottom line is to make your situations work,
    don't allow others to tell you no.
Just keep searching for resolutions in resolving the problems,
    don't give up, but choose to grow.

If one is truly industrious, zealous,
    and can work effortlessly through thick and thin,
Then keep pushing and persisting, it may add years
    to one's life. Against the game of life, you'll win.

I've been told I am an inspiring, uplifting cheerleader
    when others are in need.
Now, I've decided to direct that focus inward,
    to do it for myself, for lil' ol' me.

After reaching the point in sharing and revealing
    parts of my life in this narrative,
I no longer need to feel malcontent or sorry,
    but for my negative past to forgive.

It now gives me more freedom, and it is refreshing
    to be able to laugh and to smile.
This all leads and has guided me in having
    a much more beautiful and healthier lifestyle.

To heal ourselves, we need to find humor,
    as it is a necessary ingredient.
Even if you must pretend to laugh, you should.
    It'll help the recovery be more expedient.

Changes can't be made unless first acknowledged,
    to some absolutely nothing is funny.
Some get nervously close, give up, and quit,
    losing a personality that could be sunny.

So, if one of your friends is depressed, dejected,
    and feeling alone, and a little down,
Send a corny joke or a cartoon; draw your own,
    make them laugh somehow to get rid of their frown.

One's outlook on life is shown through asking,
    "Is your glass half full?" A trite, but insightful saying.
If not, don't sit back and sulk, make the most of it,
    get up and be ready to keep on playing.

Our life is destined whether we are aware or not.
    We all do have a personal plan.
Each one of us is even allowed to make
    our own independent choices the best we can.

If some of our unsound, poorer choices are hanging us up,
    we need to set ourselves free.
Withdraw, reflect, and ask what needs to be cleared away
    so there's new growth and fresh energy.

Even when unfortunate things happen in our lives,
    we believe it's the absolute worst.
Remember, it is not always clear.
    There's a Higher reason according to the universe.

We'll wait until we are forced to change
    when things get out of control, feeling there's no exit.
Old ways and structures must first collapse
    so we can learn truths about ourselves, then, act on it.

I believe, and feel compelled, that I'm destined
    to share my story with what I've written here.
In hopes to inspire others, in keeping their smile brighter,
    not to give up, but persevere.

As one has read, one can partially see,
    how my life is evolving. It's my destiny.
Adjusting to my diabetic life has led me
    in finding my truer identity.

Yes, I certainly do feel I've experienced
    more than my fair share of vicissitudes.
Nevertheless, I've accepted it by erasing
    most of my pessimistic attitudes.

And on occasion, it has been challenging,
    and it surely has been a very big pain.
Although, through my challenges, I keep trying hard
    to do my very best to never complain.

Dealing with my abnormal blood sugars,
    I've learned I must stay determined and persevere.
Because I know even with my fighting spirit,
    my brittleness does not seem to disappear.

It's a karmic learning process. The right attitude
    fosters a wholesome body and mind.
It's ongoing, but I strongly do foresee I'll survive,
    even being legally blind.

Therefore, I will keep an expansive mind
    and stay grounded on all levels to be healthy.
My life may improve physically, emotionally,
    spiritually, and mentally.

We do need to develop trust and blind faith,
    since God's ways are far from our understanding.
Despite all of our issues, detours, and our mistakes,
    we do hope we stay in his good standing.

Neither sight nor diabetes will impede me,
    I will put my stubbornness to good use.
As I've done in all my former competitions,
    sometimes, putting my body through much abuse.

My bulldog tenacity has been used in sports,
    now, more directed toward daily living.
In addition, I will keep appreciating my body
    after I do much forgiving.

I must detach, examine myself objectively,
    removing guilt so life may improve.
Focusing my thoughts more in the present than
    fearing the future to stay in the healthy groove.

Staying flexible and patient is a must
    as my mind and body go through these changes.
Life can be mysterious with hidden motives,
    since we don't always know what life arranges.

The vibrations beating my drum have shifted greatly.
    I'm still learning to go with the flow.
Otherwise, my toxic thoughts as well as actions
    will prevent me from being able to grow.

Instead of fighting, if I can't do it, I can't;
    or if someone needs to help, so be it.
There's too much to do in this world to quit.
    This is how life is for me today; I'm not unfit!

Therefore, identify your barriers, your obstacles,
    your blocks, what's limiting you.
Tap into your latent hidden resources–what kind of changes
    can you make? What can you do?

If one's capable of gaining wisdom, altering their attitude,
    behavior, and perceptions,
Then it will be much easier to change one's reality
    without any need for questions.

My story may widen one's eyes, sparking the light
to inner self-knowledge in what to do.
Here's hoping your journey to heal begins on such a road
to a more beautiful, healthful you.

In my story, THE BITTERSWEETNESS OF DIABETES,
every single word is true.
At least, over these trying years, it has been for me,
perhaps, not necessarily for you.

In dealing with diabetes and its complications,
I'm finding it's not such a curse.
I do feel lucky. I do feel blessed.
Leading a brittle diabetic life could be much worse.

Glossary

Access– This is prearranged transportation for those with preapproved disabilities.

Autolet– A device used to extract the blood for self-checking your glucose levels.

Basal Rate– The continuous rate or flow of insulin that is delivered in units per hour within a 24-hour period.

Bolus– An amount of insulin delivered in addition to your basal rate for the intake of food and to correct high blood glucose levels.

Brittle Diabetic– Has fluctuating blood sugars from very low below 50 to above 300 unrelated to lifestyle inconsistencies and indiscretions. The normal range is 80-120.

B.S.– My slang for blood sugar.

Cannula– A soft catheter that stays in your body that is part of an infusion set.

CGM– Continuous Glucose Monitor, a device which measures one's glucose level every five minutes. It helps to detect trends and patterns in one's glucose. It alarms if outside one's target glucose range.

Concrete Sequential– Black and white, one who needs order and is very organized, liking things in its proper place. The opposite of abstract random.

Cranefly– One of my husband's many nicknames.

Endocrinologist– A doctor who specializes in disorders of the endocrine system, such as diabetes.

Filling Needles– A sterile needle to extract the insulin from its vial to fill the cartridges for the insulin pump.

Glucagon– A substance given by injection for serious low blood sugars to help bring the person back to consciousness.

Gluco Watch G-2– An experimental device worn on the wrist to monitor blood sugars, and with an alarm that warns if too low or too high.

Glucose Control Solutions– A solution applied to a strip with your blood sugar meter to check the accuracy of its readings.

Head– Bathroom on a boat.

Hemoglobin A1Cs– A blood test taken to show an average of the last three months of your blood sugars. It also helps to predict future risks and diabetic complications. Normal for nondiabetics is 6.0; for diabetics, 7.0 or below is great.

Hyperglycemia– High blood sugar levels.

Hypoglycemia– Low blood sugar levels.

Infusion Set– A luer-lock, connector, tubing, and needle that carries insulin from the insulin pump to the user's body. There are a few varieties.

Karma– A cosmic principle based on our past actions and attitudes that can either reward or punish us in this lifetime.

Ketones– When the body can't convert the blood sugar to energy, it calls on its reserve energy supply, fat. This releases ketones into the blood, causing the blood to have high levels of acid.

Ketoacidosis– A diabetic coma where the body lacks enough insulin to break down the sugars in one's bloodstream.

Lancets– A sterile tip needle used for blood sampling in my autolet.

Larry– My husband, married on August 14, 1991.

Leash– My nickname for the tubing, part of the infusion set.

Luer-Lock– A fitting on the end of an infusion set and on the cartridge which allows them to be locked together without leaking.

Natal Chart– A map of the planets in the heavens at the exact moment, time, and place of birth.

O-rings– These are placed on the pump adapter, sealing the cartridge compartment from water.

Piston Rod– A metal threaded shaft with a cog wheel and nylon end cap that rotates by the motor of the pump, pushing the cartridge down as insulin is being used.

Pump Adapter– A device used to connect the cartridge to the infusion set to help prevent water leakage and allow air pressure to equalize.

Rapid D-6– One of three infusion sets used to attach the insulin pump to the pump user's body. It has a short tail and uses a stainless steel needle that is inserted.

Sarcoma– Malignant tumor that begins in connective tissue.

Spacey Lacy– My nickname for the treatment of soaking with lukewarm water and Epsom salt, then add aloe vera and sugar to help heal and draw out the infections on sores.

Starburst– Candy, fruit chews.

Subcutaneous– A term meaning beneath the skin.

Third Eye– When one is very intuitive or psychic, being able to pick up on things otherwise not as clear to others.

Thunder Pot– A small metal pot used as a portable toilet in the earlier days. My grandmother kept one under her bed at our cabin for convenience during the night.

Transits– The angles formed between planets in your natal chart and current planetary positions.

Type I– The pancreas works very little or not at all, thus, insulin dependent.

Type 2– Due to obesity and can be regulated by diet, pills and/or insulin.

Universe– The ultimate plan for our soul growth, the Infinite. There's no beginning or end. A realm that has no bottom or top and is limitless with assistance.

About the Author

Cheryl (Cheri) Lynn Kantzer Crane taught junior high for 22½ years, calling herself a junior high entertainer. She earned her B.A. in Education with a major in German and a minor in Physical Education, later earning her Masters in Reading and obtaining her Reading Resource Specialist degree. Near the age of 20, she was diagnosed with Type 1 diabetes. She was brittle from the onset, having unpredictable blood sugars. Despite being legally blind, she still leads a full and active life. She enjoys boating, sailing, gardening, reading, writing, and her part-time metaphysical business, Cheri's Cards & Charts, helping others find the inner light to self-knowledge. She and her husband also enjoy wintering in Arizona as "Rainbirds."

Notes

Notes

Notes

Notes

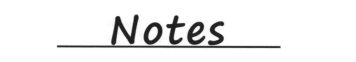

Notes

Notes

Notes

Notes